Medical
Transcription
Projects

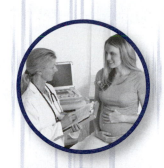
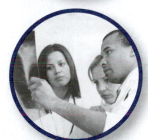
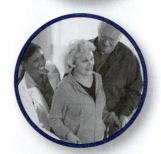
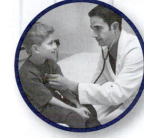
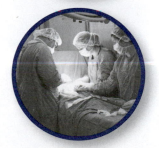

Medical Transcription Projects

DIANE M. GILMORE

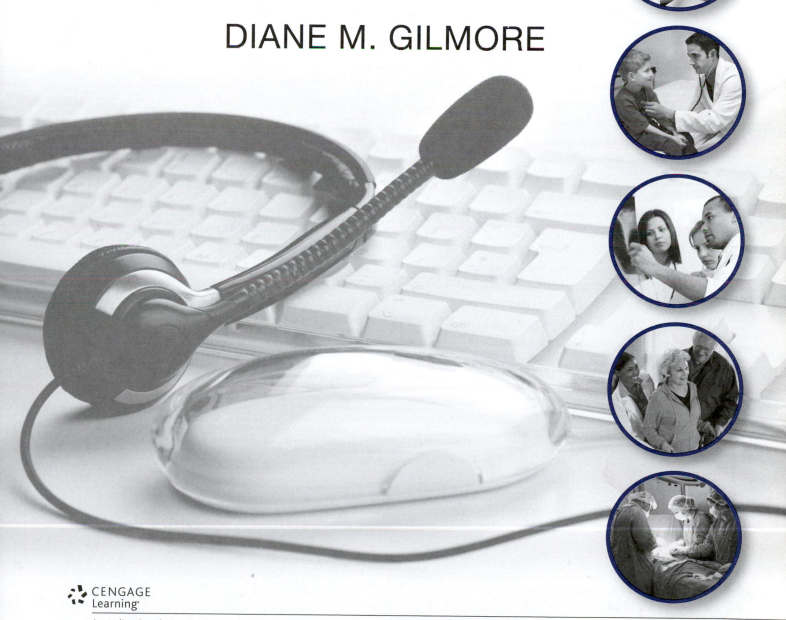

CENGAGE
Learning

Australia • Brazil • Japan • Korea • Mexico • Singapore • Spain • United Kingdom • United States

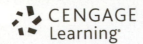

Medical Transcription Projects
Diane Gilmore

Product Director: Stephen Helba

Associate Product Manager: Christina Gifford

Senior Director, Development: Marah Bellegarde

Product Development Manager: Juliet Steiner

Senior Content Developer: Natalie Pashoukos

Product Assistant: Cassie Cloutier

Brand Manager: Wendy Mapstone

Market Development Manager: Jonathan Sheehan

Senior Production Director: Wendy A. Troeger

Production Manager: Andrew Crouth

Senior Content Project Manager: Kara A. DiCaterino

Senior Art Director: David Arsenault

Media Editor: William Overocker

Cover Images:

© iStockphoto/Michael Travers

© iStockphoto/Gene Chutka

© iStockphoto/sjlocke

© iStockphoto/kristian sekulic

© iStockphoto/Gustaf Brundin

© iStockphoto/stevecoleimages

© iStockphoto/Beyza Sultan Durna

Chapter Opener Images:

Project 1: © Sto/www.Shutterstock.com

Project 2: © pio3/www.Shutterstock.com

Project 3: © Diana Mastepanova/www
.Shutterstock.com

Project 4: © sfam_photo/www.Shutterstock.com

Project 5: © dream designs/www.Shutterstock.com

Project 6: © sfam_photo/www.Shutterstock.com

Project 7: © Sunshine Pics/www.Shutterstock.com

Project 8: © Alexonline/www.Shutterstock.com

Project 9: © Bork/www.Shutterstock.com

Project 10: © GWImages/www.Shutterstock.com

Project 11: © Alexander Tihonov/www
.Shutterstock.com

Project 12: © Tereshchenko Dmitry/www
.Shutterstock.com

Library of Congress Control Number: 2013940454

ISBN-13: 978-1-133-13289-9
ISBN-10: 1-133-13289-8

Cengage Learning
200 First Stamford Place, 4th Floor
Stamford, CT 06902
USA

Cengage Learning is a leading provider of customized learning solutions with office locations around the globe, including Singapore, the United Kingdom, Australia, Mexico, Brazil, and Japan. Locate your local office at: **www.cengage.com/global**

Cengage Learning products are represented in Canada by Nelson Education, Ltd.

To learn more about Cengage Learning, visit **www.cengage.com**

Purchase any of our products at your local college store or at our preferred online store **www.cengagebrain.com**

Notice to the Reader

Publisher does not warrant or guarantee any of the products described herein or perform any independent analysis in connection with any of the product information contained herein. Publisher does not assume, and expressly disclaims, any obligation to obtain and include information other than that provided to it by the manufacturer. The reader is expressly warned to consider and adopt all safety precautions that might be indicated by the activities described herein and to avoid all potential hazards. By following the instructions contained herein, the reader willingly assumes all risks in connection with such instructions. The publisher makes no representations or warranties of any kind, including but not limited to, the warranties of fitness for particular purpose or merchantability, nor are any such representations implied with respect to the material set forth herein, and the publisher takes no responsibility with respect to such material. The publisher shall not be liable for any special, consequential, or exemplary damages resulting, in whole or part, from the readers' use of, or reliance upon, this material.

Printed in the United States of America
1 2 3 4 5 6 7 17 16 15 14 13

TABLE OF CONTENTS

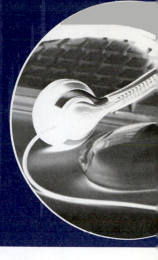

2

PROJECT 2: OPHTHALMOLOGY

3

PROJECT 3: PULMONOLOGY

4

PROJECT 4: CARDIOLOGY

5

PROJECT 5: GASTROENTEROLOGY

8

PROJECT 8: ORTHOPEDICS

9

PROJECT 9: DERMATOLOGY

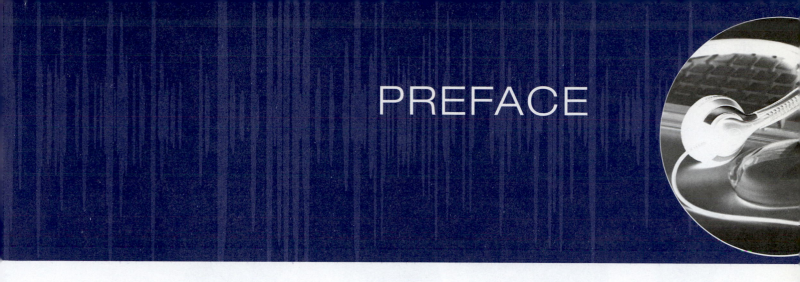

WELCOME MEMO

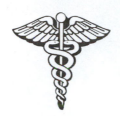

CITY MEDICAL GROUP

100 Northeast First Street, Suite 500, Nashville, TN 37204
Telephone: 615-555-0200 Fax: 615-555-0211

William Smith, MD
James A. Smith, MD
Yasmin Naimi, MD
Joseph Anderson, MD
Tiffany Benson, MD
Stephanie Soto, MD
Tina Kelly, MD

MEMORANDUM

To: Medical Transcriptionist
From: James A. Smith, MD
Subject: Welcome
Date: First Day on the Job

On behalf of the entire staff of our practice, I would like to welcome you to the City Medical Group. We are looking forward to your joining us as a new medical transcriptionist. Founded by my father, Dr. William Smith, 20 years ago, our practice provides a wide variety of medical services in different medical specialties. Our services range from family medical issues to complex medical care.

There are seven physicians in our practice, whose names are listed underneath the photo in our employee handbook. In addition, we employ various medical assistants, nurses, and front office staff. You will be called upon to perform transcription work for all of the doctors in our office. You will transcribe a variety of documents for us, including correspondence, clinic notes, consultations, history and physical exams, and operative notes, as well as radiologic and imaging findings that the physicians dictate into the patient medical record. I know you will enjoy the challenging and varied subject matter in reports you will transcribe on a daily basis.

Our goal is to provide the best medical care possible to our patients. As an employee of City Medical Group, you are now a team member of this highly respected group of physicians in the community. Again, welcome to our practice and good luck in your new job!

City Medical Group Physicians

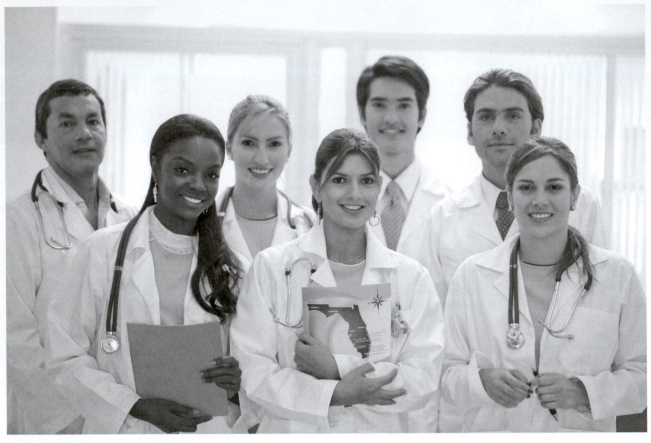

FROM LEFT TO RIGHT: William Smith, MD; Yasmin Naimi, MD; Tina Kelly MD; Tiffany Benson, MD; James A. Smith, MD; Joseph Anderson, MD; and Stephanie Soto, MD.

JOB DESCRIPTION

Job Title: Medical Transcriptionist

Required Knowledge, Skills, and Abilities:

- Knowledge of medical terminology, anatomy and physiology, clinical medicine, surgery, laboratory and imaging terminology, and terminology related to various medical specialties.

- Excellent English grammar and punctuation skills.

- Excellent listening skills.

- Knowledge of general medical documentation guidelines and practices per the Association for Healthcare Documentation Integrity (AHDI) as well as City Medical Group's in-house formatting and document guidelines.

- Ability to competently operate computer equipment, foot pedal, computer software, and medical record documentation platform used by City Medical Group.

- Understanding of and compliance with the parameters of ethical conduct, applying relevant medico-legal concepts regarding confidentiality, patient privacy, and information security as required by the Health Insurance Portability and Accountability Act (HIPAA) and Health Information Technology for Economic and Clinical Health (HITECH) Act.

Job Duties:

- Use office computer and software platform to listen to audio recordings by the physicians of City Medical Group dictating a variety of medical reports regarding our patients, including but not limited to emergency room visits, diagnostic imaging studies, operative notes, clinic notes, consultations, discharge summaries, and correspondence.

- Transcribe dictated reports and apply expert knowledge of medical terminology and medical record documentation procedures to create accurate and attractive medical reports for patient charts according to the formatting guidelines established by City Medical Group.

- Recognize, interpret, and evaluate inconsistencies in the medical dictation, edit transcribed work as necessary, and return reports in electronic form to the physician for review, correction, and/or and electronic signature for patient charts.

- Use reference materials, including the internet, appropriately and efficiently to facilitate the accuracy, clarity, and completeness of patient medical reports.

- Maintain City Medical Group's performance expectations as outlined in the Employee Handbook.

- Any other duties that may be assigned to you.

GETTING STARTED

A medical transcriptionist who can competently and accurately produce documentation pertaining to every specialty commonly encountered in the medical field is a vital team member of any successful medical transcription company or medical provider. As a medical transcriptionist, you will be expected to transcribe patient information and documentation using highly specialized language on the most up-to-date technical computer platforms and software programs. Medical Transcription Projects provides a real-life, hands-on opportunity to participate in the document-production process of a typical healthcare provider. This simulation approach enables you to practice your working knowledge of the medical reports most commonly used in hospital and ambulatory care settings. You will transcribe a variety of reports dictated by real physicians taken from reports of actual patients. Organized by body system, reports transcribed include history and physical exams, consultations, operative notes, discharge summaries, clinic notes, and radiologic studies.

Upon completion of this text, you will be able to:

- Complete terminology review exercises competently and correctly.

- Recognize missing information in a medical report and be able to insert the correct information based on the context of the report.

- Listen and edit speech-recognition-generated documents appropriately to produce a clear and accurate report according to company guidelines.

- Apply knowledge of medical terminology and rules of English grammar in the transcription and proofreading of medical dictation from real physicians using various dictation styles to produce accurate reports in a variety of medical specialties.

- Recognize, interpret, and evaluate inconsistencies in the dictation and appropriately edit, revise, and clarify the text without altering the meaning of the dictator.

- Use reference materials, including the Internet, to appropriately and efficiently locate information and use that information to produce accurate and competent medical reports.

- Format medical reports in accordance with the established guidelines of the Association for Healthcare Documentation Integrity (AHDI) and City Medical Group.

- Use computer equipment and computer software effectively and skillfully, and maintain patient files and information contained therein in accordance with confidentiality, privacy, and security guidelines.

ORGANIZATION OF TASKS

The instructions for the 12 projects in this text pertain to the types of documents produced in a wide variety of specialties encountered during a typical day of a medical transcriptionist. The first task in each project consists of "pencil" exercises to help you review the medical terminology of that specialty using a variety of methods, including multiple-choice questions, matching, and medical reading and comprehension exercises.

The second task in each project is designed to challenge your proofreading and editing skills. The proofreading exercises consist of documents that may contain errors such as missing demographic information, incorrect headings, misspelled words, or misplaced punctuation. It will be your job to read through the documents carefully and identify each error.

The third task contains two cloze exercises, which are medical reports that contain missing words. You will need to insert the correct words as you read and construct meaning from the text. The purpose of the cloze exercises is to encourage your understanding of medical terminology in the context of a medical report and to encourage you to think critically and analytically about text and content. Audio files associated with the cloze exercises are located on the Premium Website that accompanies the text at http://www.CengageBrain.com.

Tasks four and five in each project provide an opportunity for you to practice basic concepts in medical transcription and speech recognition technology (SRT). In the fourth task in each project you will transcribe dictated reports and apply expert knowledge of medical terminology and medical record documentation procedures to create accurate and attractive medical reports for patient charts.

SRT is a method whereby a physician uses a specialized computer program with a source of sound input, such as a microphone or hand-held dictation device, to interpret human speech to create a medical document. With this technology, a medical transcriptionist accesses the draft output of a report dictated by a physician through the SRT system, along with the corresponding audio file. Listening to the dictation and following along with the written draft, the medical transcriptionist makes corrections to formatting, terminology, punctuation, and grammar, and returns the edited document to the physician. The SRT reports you will access in the fifth task of each project are draft documents created by an SRT-like computer program. The documents contain errors in terminology, formatting, and other issues. You will listen to the audio file accompanying the document and make corrections to the document to create a medical report according to the guidelines of City Medical Group. Audio files associated with the transcription and SRT exercises are located on the Premium Website that accompanies the text at http://www.CengageBrain.com.

Features

Each project also includes helpful transcription tips pertaining to each medical specialty, computer tips to improve your transcription performance, and *Book of Style* tips. Various figures throughout the text illustrate the body systems covered in each project.

Helpful appendices at the back of the book provide important additional information. Appendix A includes useful medical transcription web sites; the Joint Commission's official "Do Not Use" list; and the list of Error-Prone Abbreviations, Symbols, and Dose Designations from the Institute for Safe Medication Practices (ISMP). Appendix B includes Normal Laboratory Values developed by the Medical Council of Canada (MCC) and a list of commonly used metric system units, symbols, and prefixes from the U.S. Metric Association. Appendix C presents sample reports and Appendix D includes a student progress sheet that can be used to log and monitor your progress in the course.

ADDITIONAL RESOURCES

Instructor Resources

Online Instructor Resources | ISBN-13: 978-1-133-13291-2

The instructor resources include an instructor's manual with answers to the review questions at the beginning of each project as well as the solutions to the cloze exercises, transcription exercises, and SRT exercises in each project.

Student Resources

Premium Website Printed Access Card (PAC) | ISBN-13: 978-1-285-73538-2

The Premium Website contains streaming audio files for the cloze, transcription, and SRT exercises. It also includes the accompanying student documents for the cloze exercises where you will insert the missing words for the medical reports and the SRT reports which you will correct for errors such as terminology, formatting, and spelling.

Premium Website Instant Access Code (IAC) | ISBN-13: 978-1-285-73536-8

The Premium Website contains streaming audio files for the cloze, transcription, and SRT exercises. It also includes the accompanying student documents for the cloze exercises where you will insert the missing words for the medical reports and the SRT reports which you will correct for errors such as terminology, formatting, and spelling.

Redeeming an Access Code

1. GO TO: http://www.CengageBrain.com.

2. ENTER the access code in the field, "Enter Product Access Code or Course Key."

3. REGISTER as a new user or LOG IN as an existing user if you already have an account with Cengage Learning or CengageBrain.com.

4. You will be directed to the My Home page of your account. The materials you have registered are loaded into your account and you may launch your resource by clicking the OPEN button next to the resource you would like to use.

TRANSCRIPTION INSTRUCTIONS

You will transcribe medical reports and correspondence from audio files located on the Premium Website at www .CengageBrain.com. Your goal is to produce documents with as few errors as possible. Unless otherwise specified by your instructor, review and follow these guidelines for transcribing the medical reports:

1. Become familiar with the content and format of the sample forms provided for you and the formatting guidelines of City Medical Group.

2. Open Microsoft (MS) Word. Go to the Premium Website and locate the audio file of the report to be transcribed, then listen to the dictation and transcribe each report. Do not insert a heading into the document if the text requires a second page, but let the text wrap naturally to the second page and continue typing. Transcribe the reports using the formatting guidelines provided in this book.

3. When you are finished transcribing a report, proofread your work and save the document to your student blank CD disk or pursuant to the instructions for saving your work by your instructor using the last name of the patient. If there is more than one patient with the same last name, save the document with a slightly different name; for example, HENDERSON and HENDERSON1. If desired, you may include an indication of the type of document in the file name, as follows:

   CN: clinic note
   HP: history and physical
   OP: operative note
   CN: consultation
   DS: discharge summary
   LT: letter
   For example, HENDERSON.CN or HENDERSON1.HP.

   You may also organize the files on your CD or other area where student data is saved by project name and/or number. When you begin a new project, create a folder on your CD for all of the documents in that project by name or project number; for example, PROJECT 4 or CARDIOLOGY. Now all of the work from that project can be contained in its respective folder.

3. Type the report verbatim, or word for word, although light editing is acceptable to correct the physician's grammatical errors or errors in context. If you encounter a word you cannot understand, use the reference resources available to you (e.g., medical dictionary, word books, the Internet) to try and find the word. If you still cannot understand the word after reasonable research, leave a blank of seven spaces using the underline key (_____) in that portion of the dictation and flag that portion of the report.

4. You may use abbreviations in the body of the report as dictated by the physician. Do not use an abbreviation in preoperative or postoperative diagnosis sections of an operative note or in the admitting or discharge diagnosis sections of a discharge summary. You may use laboratory abbreviations in these areas to make the report more easily readable (such as "INR" versus "internal normalized ratio"). Do not expand an abbreviation unless you are absolutely sure of its meaning.

5. Refer to the Joint Commission's and the ISMP's respective lists of abbreviations, acronyms, symbols, and medication dosages that should not be used in reports due to the potential for them to be misread or misunderstood, located in Appendix A. For the reports in this textbook, make the appropriate term or medication dosage substitution when you hear one of these terms dictated.

6. Transcribe the text as dictated into the appropriate headings, in paragraph form, according to the samples in this book and the formatting guidelines of City Medical Group. If additional headings are dictated, they should be typed with the same formatting and capitalization as the rest of the headings in the report. See the formatting guidelines for more information.

7. If the physician dictates the word "same" for a postoperative diagnosis in an operative report (indicating it is the same text as the preoperative diagnosis), do not type the word "same." Instead, type the same text as in the preoperative diagnosis.

8. When typing dates, follow the dictator's style. If the dictator uses numeric dates, use two digits for the day and month and four digits for the year (01/01/xxxx). If the dictator uses text for the date (January 10, 20xx), transcribe the date in that format.

9. Decision-making and critical-thinking skills are important for a medical transcriptionist. You will be required to make formatting and editing decisions regarding the documents you produce. The final report must be complete, accurate, and grammatically correct by medical office standards. Listen for inconsistencies you may encounter in the dictation, such as numbered items dictated out of order, mispronounced words, and other possible dictation errors. These inconsistencies have been intentionally dictated into some reports to give you practice in listening closely to details. If you can resolve the inconsistency confidently and competently (such as number items in correct chronological order, or knowing the patient, Mary, is female and not male), then edit the report accordingly. However, if you cannot resolve the discrepancy with certainty, insert a blank so that it may be brought to the attention of your instructor for clarification.

10. When you are finished with a report, print one copy for your instructor and save the completed document to your disk in the method outlined above or that is preferred by your instructor for saving documents on your CD. Your instructor will provide you with feedback on the quality of your work in each project.

11. Use the Student Progress Sheet in this book to log and monitor your progress in the course.

DOCUMENT FORMATTING GUIDELINES

The following are the formatting guidelines for preparing documents for City Medical Group. These rules are based on company preference as well as *The Book of Style for Medical Transcription, 3rd ed.*, by the Association for Healthcare Documentation Integrity (AHDI).

General Transcription Guidelines

All documents are to be typed in MS Word using <u>Times New Roman 12-point</u> font using <u>1-inch margins</u> on all sides of the page. The title of the document is centered at the top of the page in all caps, with no bold or underlining. The text of the report begins two lines under the title, single-spaced. The text should be <u>left justified</u> with a ragged right margin. Do not indent any paragraphs. Do not bold, underline, or italicize anything in the report. Do not use the Tab key; use two spaces instead. Double-space between paragraphs.

Transcribe the text as dictated. Try not to change what the dictator says if at all possible. Only change the dictation if it is grammatically incorrect or factually wrong (such as he dictates "he" instead of "she"). For example, if the dictator says "nonicteric," don't change it to "anicteric" for style's sake. The same with "a half" or "one-half." Type what is dictated.

It is permissible to lightly edit to fix an awkward construction of a sentence, though this is not often necessary). For example, a doctor might dictate, "She has both feet ulcerations." You should transcribe that as "She has ulcerations on both feet." You haven't changed what the doctor said, simply rearranged the words to be better understood by anyone reading the transcription.

Examples of some other instances where an MT would be expected to edit include:

- The patient was seen by **me** (not myself).

- In **regard** (not regards) to this patient.

- Dr. Jones **and I** will continue to manage this patient (not I and Dr. Jones; me and Dr. Jones; Dr. Jones and me; or Dr. Jones and myself).

- When the doctor refers to a male patient as "she" or female patient as "he."

- When the sentence is grammatically incorrect in terms of tense or plural versus singular: "The x-rays **reveals** a fracture." "The patient's mother and father **is** in the room." Change the erroneous text so that subjects agree with verbs.

- When a doctor dictates run-on sentences. "She came to the hospital with symptoms of chest pain, shortness of breath, her white count was elevated." Place a transitional word between the clauses or separate the clauses into two independent clauses: "She came to the hospital with symptoms of chest pain, shortness of breath, **and** her white count was elevated." or separate into two sentences: "She came to the hospital with chest pain **and** shortness of breath. **Her** white count was elevated."

Abbreviations, Brief Forms and Slang Terms

You may abbreviate within the body of the report. However, please spell out abbreviations in the DIAGNOSIS, IMPRESSION, and PROCEDURES sections of the report, even if an abbreviation is dictated. Some abbreviations are acceptable and even preferred to make the report more readable, such as Pap smear, INR, labs, IV, MRI, CT, and some other lab terms.

Do not use contractions in the medical report (can't, don't, I'll, etc.) unless it is part of a direct quote.

Many brief forms are acceptable. Brief forms used in lab words should be expanded to better delineate their meanings. Below is a list of some common dictated brief forms and slang that should be transcribed:

Brief Form/Slang	Expand To
alk phos	alkaline phosphatase
echo	echocardiogram
postop	postoperative; postoperatively
preop	preoperative; preoperatively
temp	temperature
appy	appendectomy
bili	bilirubin
crit	hematocrit
lytes	electrolytes
chem	chemistry (unless a name brand test like Chem-7)
meds	medications
vanc	vancomycin
gent	gentamicin
amp	ampule or ampicillin
bicarb	bicarbonate
sat	saturation (as in oxygen saturation)
exlap	exploratory laparotomy

Allergies

Positive allergies should be typed in all caps two spaces after the heading.

    ALLERGIES: IBUPROFEN.
    ALLERGIES: Skin rash to NAFCILLIN.

Apostrophes

Do not use apostrophes with medical eponyms: He presented with a Hartmann pouch. This patient has Down syndrome with early onset of Alzheimer disease. Not Hartmann's pouch, Down's syndrome, or Alzheimer's disease.

Unless the dictator indicates a direct quote, do not type contractions: don't, didn't, couldn't, can't. Type in full: do not, did not, could not, cannot.

Blanks

If you cannot understand what the dictator is saying, leave a blank consisting of seven (7) underscores for the blank.

Dates

Generally, type dates as dictated with a comma following the year if the date is within a sentence. Use ordinals when the day of the month precedes the month and is preceded by *the*; do not use commas. Do not use ordinals in month/day/year format.

> the 10th of May, not May 10th, 20XX

Genus and Species Names

Type a genus name (e.g., staphylococcus) in lowercase letters when used alone. Capitalize the genus name when it is accompanied by its species name (e.g., Staphylococcus aureus). Use lowercase letters when genus names are used in plural and adjectival forms and when used in the vernacular; for example, when they stand alone (without a species name).

> staphylococci
> staphylococcal infection
> staph infection
> strep throat

Headings

Major section headings as well as subheadings are all caps with a colon (:). Do not bold the headings. Type the text two spaces after the heading. Double space between major sections of the report. If most headings are dictated within the report but some are missing, please add a heading or subheading for clarity.

Although the sample reports provided for you illustrate standard headings to use, the physician may use a different heading. In that case, transcribe headings as dictated unless they are clearly incorrect, like a review of systems for the physical examination. You may add a heading if one is not dictated but do not take text out of order or move the text around just for the sake of adding a heading where none is dictated. You should follow the dictator's lead in the transcription of headings. It is permissible to change a heading name slightly to match what the dictator says, or add headings if the physician dictates a heading that is not on the samples provided. Change the headings to match what is dictated. For example, if the sample report provided says "Admission Diagnosis" and the dictator says "Admitting Diagnoses," then you may change this. Likewise, if you need to show that current medications, or home medications, or preadmission medications are being dictated, for example, then you might type "Current Medications," "Home Medications," etc., to accurately reflect what the dictator means.

Joint Commission Dangerous Abbreviations and ISMP List

Our practice conforms with Joint Commission recommendations and the ISMP List of Error-Prone Abbreviations, Symbols, and Dose Designations. Please consult these lists when transcribing these abbreviations.

Medications

If more than one medication is listed, they should be transcribed in a vertical list. Even if the information is given in a general list format without dosages, place them in a numbered list with the number placed at the left margin, followed by two spaces. Let the text wrap naturally to the next line and do not try to line up the text using the Tab key.

If the doctor dictates a little introduction, like "This patient's current medications include"—do not type this. Instead, change the heading to Current Medications, Transfer Medications, Admission Medications, etc., if that describes what the doctor is saying. Do not use Word's auto numbering function for numbered lists. Begin the list on the line below the heading with no extra space below the heading. Type the number at the left margin, followed by two spaces and the name of the medication.

MEDICATIONS

1. (space)(space)Lisinopril 10 mg daily.
2. (space)(space)Altace.

Military Time

Sometimes physicians use military time instead of clock time. Transcribe this using four digits with no colon. The word "hours" may be added for clarity.

12:00 midnight	0000 hours	12:00 noon	1200 hours
01:00 a.m.	0100 hours	01:00 p.m.	1300 hours
02:00 a.m.	0200 hours	02:00 p.m.	1400 hours
03:00 a.m.	0300 hours	03:00 p.m.	1500 hours
04:00 a.m.	0400 hours	04:00 p.m.	1600 hours
05:00 a.m.	0500 hours	05:00 p.m.	1700 hours
06:00 a.m.	0600 hours	06:00 p.m.	1800 hours
07:00 a.m.	0700 hours	07:00 p.m.	1900 hours
08:00 a.m.	0800 hours	08:00 p.m.	2000 hours
09:00 a.m.	0900 hours	09:00 p.m.	2100 hours
10:00 a.m.	1000 hours	10:00 p.m.	2200 hours
11:00 a.m.	1100 hours	11:00 p.m.	2300 hours

Numbers

Use arabic numbers exclusively except when an object of a sentence or when implying a precise quantity where none is intended.

> The patient was injured 1 time previously.
> The patient has 1 brother in the Navy.

BUT:

> If one looks closely, a fracture can be seen on the x-ray.
> His symptoms went from one extreme to the other.

> She is the one who is getting the surgery done today.
> I looked inside one of the charts for the information.

Note that some items may start with an arabic number and this is acceptable. For example, in operative notes, the anesthesia, drains or blood loss headings often start with a number and is acceptable and preferred.

> ANESTHESIA: 1% Marcaine
> ESTIMATED BLOOD LOSS: 30 mL.

In most cases (especially with a patient's age), however, try not to start out a sentence with a number. Add an article or a word before it.

Ordinal numbers (1st, 2nd, 3rd, etc.) can be written out from first to ninth. For ordinal number 10th and above, use arabic numbers.

List more than one item in a section (such as diagnoses, medications, or procedures) in a numbered list beneath the heading. Type the number and two spaces after the period. Do not number the past medical history or past surgical history sections unless they are dictated that way. Let the text wrap naturally to the next line and do not try to line up the text using the Tab key.

Spell out nonspecific (indefinite) numeric expressions.

> She described hundreds of symptoms. *(not 100s)*
> I believe several thousand people were tested.

Physical Examination and Review of Systems

The heading PHYSICAL EXAMINATION is typed in all caps, flush left, followed by a colon, and the text begins two spaces thereafter. The text is typed in one paragraph. Subheadings are typed in all caps, followed by a colon, and the text begins two spaces thereafter. Do not use bold.

> PHYSICAL EXAMINATION: VITAL SIGNS: Temperature 100.2, pulse 140, respiratory rate 24, and weight 130 pounds. GENERAL: The patient is a well-nourished female in no apparent distress, who is mostly cooperative with the exam. HEENT: No facial asymmetry. NECK: No masses or lymphadenopathy. LUNGS: Clear to auscultation. HEART: Regular rate and rhythm. ABDOMEN: Soft and nontender. EXTREMITIES: No edema. NEUROLOGIC: The patient is grossly intact.

The heading REVIEW OF SYSTEMS is typed in all caps and flush left. The text is typed in paragraph form, headings in all caps, not bolded.

> REVIEW OF SYSTEMS: CONSTITUTIONAL: No fevers. No chills. EYES: No blurry vision. No discharge. EARS, NOSE, AND THROAT: No external discharge. No mucous membrane thrush. CARDIOVASCULAR: No chest pain. No palpitations. RESPIRATORY: No cough. No sputum. GASTROINTESTINAL: No nausea. No vomiting. No diarrhea. GENITOURINARY: No hematuria, frequency, or dysuria. MUSCULOSKELETAL: No arthralgias, myalgias, or joint deformities. NEUROLOGIC: No focal weakness. No evidence of seizure.

Sometimes the physician will dictate the physical exam or review of systems in a narrative form without any headings whatsoever. In this case, follow his/her lead and transcribe the text without headings. However, if the physician uses one heading, you must insert all the other headings for uniformity.

Symbols

Do not use superscripts, subscripts, or the degrees sign in a medical report. You can use the percent sign when preceded by a number, as well as other symbols such as:

> / ( ) + − & $ # ! @

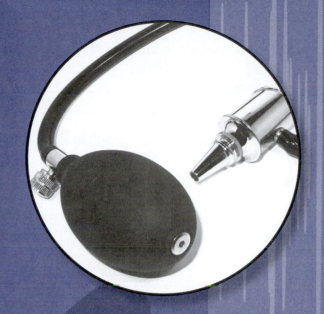

PROJECT 1

Otorhinolaryngology

TASK 1-1A: TRUE/FALSE EXERCISES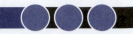

Instructions: Read each statement and indicate whether it is true or false. If false, rewrite the sentence to make the statement true, replacing either the italicized term or the description/definition of the term contained in the sentence.

1. Statement: *Otitis media* is an infection of the nares.

   Answer: _____

   Correction, if false: _____

   _____

2. Statement: The laryngeal system is involved in the detection of *sound*.

   Answer: _____

   Correction, if false: _____

   _____

3. Statement: A broken nose will result in a *deviated septum*.

   Answer: _____

   Correction, if false: _____

   _____

4. Statement: The word *sinus* generally means a cavity within a bone.

   Answer: _____

   Correction, if false: _____

   _____

5. Statement: Another name for ear wax is *cerumen*.

   Answer: _____

   Correction, if false: _____

   _____

6. Statement: A *laparoscope* is used to examine the ear and tympanic membrane.

   Answer: _____

   Correction, if false: _____

   _____

7. Statement: The outer or external portion of the ear is called the *pinna*.

   Answer: _____

   Correction, if false: _____

   _____

8. Statement: IU is the abbreviation for *both ears*.

   Answer: _____

   Correction, if false: _____

   _____

9. **Statement:** The medical term for the voice box is the *epiglottis*.
   Answer: _____
   Correction, if false: _____
   _____

10. **Statement:** In the physical exam, the abbreviation HEENT stands for *head, eyes, ears, neck, and throat*.
    Answer: _____
    Correction, if false: _____
    _____

11. **Statement:** The stapes is part of the anatomy of the *throat*.
    Answer: _____
    Correction, if false: _____
    _____

12. **Statement:** The *maxillary* sinuses are located in the cheeks.
    Answer: _____
    Correction, if false: _____
    _____

13. **Statement:** A cochlear implant is a surgical repair of the *tympanic membrane*.
    Answer: _____
    Correction, if false: _____
    _____

14. **Statement:** A *polysomnography* measures a patient's hearing.
    Answer: _____
    Correction, if false: _____
    _____

15. **Statement:** Age-related hearing loss is called *presbycusis*.
    Answer: _____
    Correction, if false: _____
    _____

TASK 1-1B: COMBINING FORMS EXERCISES ● ● ●

Instructions: Write the meaning of the following combining forms.

1. cochle/o _____

2. pharyng/o _____

3. palat/o _____

4. audit/o _____

5. ethm/o _____

6. turbin/o _____

7. tympan/o _____

8. gloss/o _____

9. nas/o _____

10. bucc/o _____

11. sphen/o _____

12. sept/o _____

13. tonsill/o _____

14. aden/o _____

15. acous/o _____

TASK 1-1C: MEDICAL COMPREHENSION EXERCISE

Instructions: Read the clinic note below and answer the questions that follow by choosing the correct letter answer.

SUBJECTIVE: The patient is a 29-year-old male who has complained of sinus congestion and is returning for followup of his bronchitis. He has been using Afrin nasal spray more than the prescribed dose. The patient has been giving himself 2 doses 4-5 times a day. He has been told of the side effects of Afrin abuse. The patient was counseled about his blood pressure of 160/94, especially in view of his family history. He was given the option of following a diet or going on blood pressure medication. He chose the diet and weight loss at this time.

OBJECTIVE: Vital signs: Blood pressure 160/94, weight 205. ENT: Ears clear, pharynx without erythema, nares erythematous. There is no sinus tenderness. Heart: S1 and S2, no murmurs, rubs, or gallops. Lungs: Rales are heard at the bases without wheezes. Extremities: No clubbing, cyanosis, or edema.

ASSESSMENT: 1. Rule out right lower lobe pneumonia. 2. Afrin abuse.

PLAN: Chest x-ray, erythromycin 250 mg p.o. q.i.d. for 10 days, Vancenase AQ 2 puffs in each nostril b.i.d., lipid panel, chemistry panel, and Hismanal 1 tablet p.o. daily. The patient was given dietary information for controlling cholesterol and reducing sodium intake. He will return in 2 weeks for followup.

1. What is Afrin?
   A. A corticosteroid used to reduce inflammation
   B. An antibiotic
   C. A nasal spray used to relieve congestion
   D. A bronchodilator used to clear nasal passages

2. Why does the physician discuss the patient's blood pressure with him?
   A. It is too low.
   B. It is too high.
   C. It is stable.
   D. He wanted to review the patient's family history with him.

3. The nares are erythematous, which means
   A. they are clear.
   B. they are swollen.
   C. they are boggy.
   D. they are reddened.

4. How many times per day is the patient to take his antibiotic?
   A. Four times
   B. Two times
   C. Three times
   D. One time

5. Rales in the lungs sound like
   A. whistling.
   B. rattling.
   C. thumping.
   D. snoring.

6. In the Plan, why would the physician order a lipid panel?
   A. To review the patient's cholesterol, HDL, and LDL values
   B. To review the patient's blood sugar
   C. To review the patient's blood pressure
   D. To review the patient's sodium intake

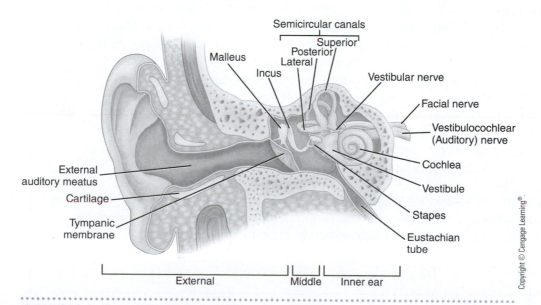

FIGURE 1-1 Outer, Middle, and Inner Ear Structures

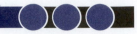

TASK 1-2:   PROOFREADING EXERCISES

Instructions: The proofreading documents below are designed to challenge your proofreading and editing skills. The documents may contain missing demographic information, incorrect headings, misspelled words, misplaced punctuation, and other errors within the document. Read each report below and identify the error by circling the word. Then retype the document with the corrected text and formatting. When finished, proofread your work and save the document to your student disk using a different file name.

PROOFREADING EXERCISE 1

CHIEF COMPLAINT: Dysphasia.

HISTORY OF PRESENT ILLNESS: This is a 67-year old male with a history of a left vocal cord cancer, which was treated with radiation therapy, he subsequently had recurrence, which resulted in hemilaryngectomy. After that, he had another primary requiring total laryngectomy. Then he developed a radiation induced sarcoma of the nasopharynx and, therefore, underwent resection of this with reconstruction with a pectoralis flap. His postoperative course was complicated by necrosis and fistula, with the requirement of being taken back to the operating room for a second operation last month for debredement and reclosure of the wound.

Today he is here for follow up. He recently underwent an esophageal dilation and he reports a 40 percent improvement in his swallowing since that time. He reports dysphagia for solids and liquids, which has been worsening since his dilation. He denies any dyspnea, odynophagia, otalgia, weight loss, or any other complains.

Past medical history, past surgical history, medications, allergies, family history, social history, and review of systems were reviewed and found to be unchanged from the previous note.

PHYSICAL EXAMINATION: Vital signs are as follows: Temperature 96.9, pulse 57, respiratory rate 16, and weight 154 pounds, blood pressure 104-50. In general, the patient is a well-nourished male in no apparent distress, alert and oriented times 3. Voice is with an electrolarynx. Head: No scalp or facial lesions or asymmetry. Eyes: Extraocular movements intact. Inicteric. Ears: TMs intact with no middle ear efusions. Nose: No masses. No discharge. Septum is straight. Orocavity/oropharynx: Mucous membranes are moist. By visualization and palpation, no masses or lesions are seen including cheeks, floor of mouth hard and soft palate, tongue, tonsils, posterior pharynx, lips, teeth, and gums. Indirect laryngoscopy: No masses within the nasopharynx, and the pectoralis flap is visible and viable. Neck: Laryngectomy stoma is widely patient without any lesions. There are no neck masses or lymphadenopathy. Incisions are all well heeled.

IMPRESSION: No evidence of disease at this time. Patient does have worsening dysphagia and was offered esophageal dilation whenever he desires it. He does not want any at this time and would like to return to clinic in three months.

PLAN: Return to clinic in 3 months.

PROOFREADING EXERCISE 2

Dear Doctor Peterson:

I saw your patient Haley Jones in my clinic today. As you recall, the patient is a 49-year-old female with snoring, nasal congestion, and acute sinusitis. She had a sleep study performed, which showed no apneas. She just has snoring without any apneic episodes, she also recently has had an acute sinus infection, which you have treated with cefuroxime. She reports the antibiotic is improving her symptoms. Previously I had her on Flonaze, Astelin, and normal saline irrigation. She reports moderate compliant with this and reports some benefit from these treatments but is not satisfied with the results.

On physical exam, I note that the left side of her nose continues to be congested and the right side is clear today. She has a moderate sized soft plate with a long uvula.

I have recommended finishing the antibiotics and maximizing her medical therapy with the nasal sprays and normal saline irrigation. We have ordered a ct scan to evaluate her sinuses for chronic sinusitis. For the snoring, I have recommended radiofrequency stiffening of her palate with possible trimming of her uvula in order to improve her snoring. I have told her that this will likely require 2-3 treatments to cure her of her snoring. These are in office treatments that take approximately 1 hour for each treatment session. She will consider this and will notify me if she is interested. I have aksed her to return to my clinic after completing the CT scan.

Thankyou for allowing me to participate in the care of this patient. If you have any questions, please do not hesitate to call.

Sincerely,

Mike Yao, MD

 OTORHINOLARYNGOLOGY TRANSCRIPTION **TIPS**

1. The abbreviations *AD, AS,* and *AU,* stand for *aurus dextra* (right ear), *aurus sinistra* (left ear), and *aures uterque* (both ears). However, the Institute for Safe Medication Practices (ISMP) has included these abbreviations among those that are frequently misinterpreted and involved in harmful medication errors. You should expand these abbreviations when used in general narrative, but they can be abbreviated when transcribing information associated with diagnostic testing and measured values. To be sure, check with your employer as to the company's policy about transcribing these abbreviations.

2. Many physicians mistakenly refer to the term *nare* when talking about one nostril. The correct term is *naris,* and the term *nares* refers to both nostrils of the nose.

3. Remember, the *malleus* is one of three auditory ossicles in the middle ear. Do not type the word *malleolus,* which is the rounded bony prominence of the ankle joint.

4. When transcribing diagnostic studies related to the ears, do not confuse the abbreviations *EMG* and *ENG. EMG* is the abbreviation for *electromyelography,* which is a test used by neurologists to

evaluate abnormal nerve function. *ENG* stands for *electronystagmography*, which is a test used by audiologists to evaluate balance and movement disorders.

5. When transcribing ENT reports, pay attention to the anatomy referred to by the dictator. *Aural*, a term relating to the ear, sounds very similar to *oral*, a term relating to the mouth.

TASK 1-3:   CLOZE EXERCISES

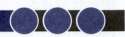

Instructions: The audio files for the following cloze exercises are located on the Premium Website that accompanies this text (ISBN-13: 978-1-285-73537-5) at http://www.CengageBrain.com. If this is the first time you are registering your account, see the Preface for further instructions.

Once you are logged in to your account, locate the dictation file and Word document for the following cloze exercises. Open the audio file to be reviewed according to the exercise number indicated, along with its corresponding Word document. Listen to the dictation and read along with the text, filling in the missing words in the report by thinking critically and analytically about the context of the text you are reading. When finished, proofread your work and save the document according to your instructor's directions.

CLOZE EXERCISE 1: Clinic Note_Report 6182
Patient Name: Evan Jones
Medical Record Number: 91264

CLOZE EXERCISE 2: Clinic Note_Report 6103
Patient Name: Sandra Wells
Medical Record Number: 06668

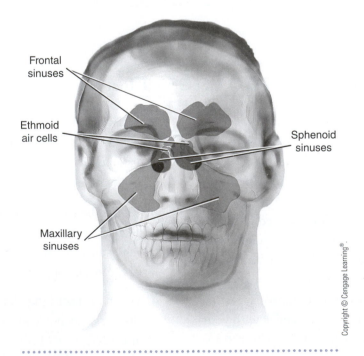

Frontal sinuses

Ethmoid air cells

Sphenoid sinuses

Maxillary sinuses

FIGURE 1-2 Frontal View of the Paranasal Sinuses

TASK 1-4: TRANSCRIPTION EXERCISES

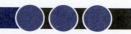

Instructions: The audio files for the following transcription exercises are located on the Premium Website that accompanies this text (ISBN-13: 978-1-285-73537-5) at http://www.CengageBrain.com. If this is the first time you are registering your account, see the Preface for further instructions.

Once you are logged in to your account, locate and open the audio file to be transcribed according to the exercise number indicated and transcribe each report. Do not insert a heading into the document if the text requires a second page, but let the text wrap naturally to the second page and continue typing. Transcribe the reports using the formatting specifics indicated in the Document Formatting Guidelines located at the beginning of this book. When finished, proofread your work and save the document according to your instructor's directions.

TRANSCRIPTION EXERCISE 1: Clinic Note_Report 6142

Patient Name: Anna Guzman
Medical Record Number: 89806

TRANSCRIPTION EXERCISE 2: Clinic Note_Report 6119

Patient Name: Jeremiah Coleman
Medical Record Number: 38392

TRANSCRIPTION EXERCISE 3: Procedure Note_Report 6146

Patient Name: Gustavo Chavez
Medical Record Number: 67343

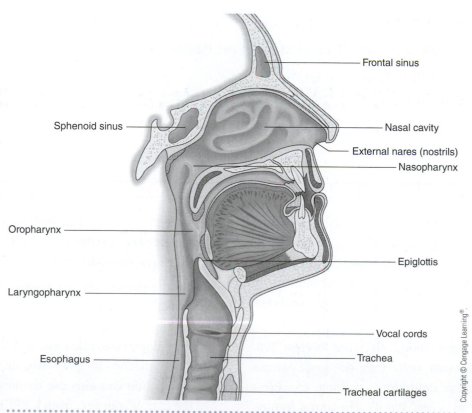

FIGURE 1-3 Sagittal View of the Nasopharynx, Oropharynx, and Laryngopharynx

TRANSCRIPTION EXERCISE 4: Operative Report_Report 6171

Patient Name: Timothy Hall
Medical Record Number: 53196

TRANSCRIPTION EXERCISE 5: Letter_Report 6114

Patient Name: Catava Boro
Medical Record Number: 06114

TASK 1-5: SPEECH RECOGNITION EXERCISES
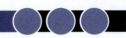

Instructions: The audio files for the following speech recognition exercises are located on the Premium Website that accompanies this text (ISBN-13: 978-1-285-73537-5) at http://www.CengageBrain.com. If this is the first time you are registering your account, see the Preface for further instructions.

Once you are logged in to your account, locate the dictation file and Word document for the following speech recognition exercises. Open the audio file to be reviewed according to the exercise number indicated, along with its corresponding Word document. Listen to the dictation and read along with the text, making corrections to the text with regard to formatting, terminology, grammar, spelling, and punctuation. When finished, proofread your work and save the document according to your instructor's directions.

SRT EXERCISE 1: Clinic Note_Report 13

Patient Name: Dennis Hill
Medical Record Number: 22930

SRT EXERCISE 2: Clinic Note_Report 21

Patient Name: Allan Cook
Medical Record Number: 87434

SRT EXERCISE 3: Middle Ear MRI and MRA of the Posterior Fossa Vasculature_Report 7

SRT EXERCISE 4: Clinic Note_Report 7

Patient Name: Cindy Ross
Medical Record Number: 23309

 COMPUTER SOFTWARE **TIPS**

1. If you make a mistake while transcribing (like accidentally deleting blocks of text), on the **Quick Access** tool bar, choose the **UNDO** button or press **CTRL + Z**. You can use this feature repeatedly to backtrack through and undo the most recent editing changes (or mistakes) you made.

2. In the **Proofing** section, select the **Review Tab**, then the **Research** button to do some simple research, such as definitions, spelling, etc. Press **SHIFT + F7** to access Word's Thesaurus feature.

Type in any word you wish to look up and press the little green arrow to the right of the search box to see synonyms for your word.

3. On the **Home Tab**, the **Font** section has a button that allows you to automatically change the case of highlighted text. Options are sentence case, lowercase, uppercase, title case, and toggle case, which automatically changes what you have to the opposite. You can also use the keyboard to change the case of your text from UPPER to lower to First

Letters Capitalized by highlighting the text with the mouse, then holding down **SHIFT** and F3 keys to cycle through these options.

4. You can open more than one document at once by selecting several files in the Open dialog box. For noncontiguous files, click on the first file and then press **CTRL + CLICK** for subsequent files. For contiguous files in the list, click on the first file and press **SHIFT + CLICK** on the last file. Then press the Open button to open all of the files.

5. Press **CTRL + S** to quickly save your document without taking your hands away from the keyboard to use the mouse.

 ## GENERAL BOOK OF STYLE **TIPS**

1. Do not use a period in most abbreviations.

HPI	history of present illness
RN	registered nurse
ED	emergency department

Other abbreviations do use a period, such as with *Dr.* or *Mr.*, and some medical abbreviations, such as *p.r.n.*

> Dr. Smith will be out of the office until Friday.
> The patient is to take lactulose p.r.n. for constipation.

Note: While the use of periods in abbreviated personal and courtesy titles is still acceptable, there continues to be a strong trend toward dropping them. Be sure to check facility preference.

2. Capitalize the first word following the first set of opening quotation marks in directly quoted speech.

> The division clerk said, "I was late to work today."

However, do not capitalize the second part of an interrupted sentence in a quotation:

> "The nursing staff reported no new events last night," said Dr. Jones, "after the patient was given a sedative for sleep."

3. Physicians often use the word *reoccur* in dictation. There is actually no such word as *reoccur*, so you should edit it to the correct term, *recur*.

> Dictated (incorrect): The patient had no reoccurrence of her seizures.
> Transcribed (correct): The patient had no recurrence of her seizures.

4. Medical transcriptionists often mistranscribe the term *follow up* in medical reports. Use the words *follow up* and *followup* correctly according to context. Use *followup* for the noun and adjectival forms. Use *follow up* as two words only when the word is used as a verb or action word.

> The patient has a followup appointment with us next week.
> The patient will be getting followup labs tomorrow.
> The patient will follow up with her cardiologist after discharge.

5. Avoid the frequent mistranscriptions of the word *alot*, *alright*, and *often times*. The correct terms are *a lot*, *all right*, and *oftentimes*.

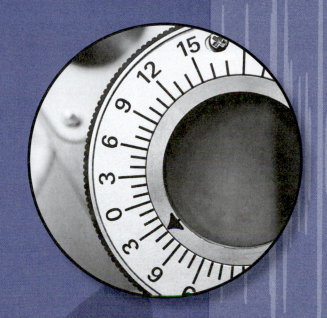

PROJECT 2

Ophthalmology

TASK 2-1A: MATCHING EXERCISE

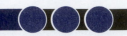

Instructions: Match the following ophthalmologic disorders in the left column with their corresponding definitions in the right column. Use each definition only once.

Term	Definition
1. _____ keratitis	a. Inflammation of the conjunctiva caused by bacteria, a virus, or fungi.
2. _____ strabismus	b. The blockage of the meibomian gland with oil secretion.
3. _____ blepharitis	c. The growth of conjunctival tissue over the cornea.
4. _____ trichiasis	d. Extreme sensitivity to light.
5. _____ xanthelasma	e. The chronic inflammation of the lid margins.
6. _____ iridoplegia	f. Inflammation of the cornea of the eye.
7. _____ pterygium	g. Impaired vision caused by old age.
8. _____ glaucoma	h. A condition in which the eyelashes grow inward and rub the cornea of the eye.
9. _____ myopia	i. The abnormal outward curling of the eyelid away from the globe.
10. _____ photophobia	j. A yellow, fatty spot or bump on the inner corner of the upper eyelid, the lower eyelid, or both eyelids.
11. _____ nyctalopia	k. Poor vision in reduced light or at night ("night blindness").
12. _____ presbyopia	l. Paralysis of the iris.
13. _____ conjunctivitis	m. A condition in which the eyes cannot focus on the same target simultaneously under normal conditions ("cross eyes").
14. _____ ectropion	n. An optic condition in which light rays are improperly focused in front of the retina, resulting in blurred vision ("nearsightedness").
15. _____ chalazion	o. A disease of the eye that causes damage to the optic nerve.

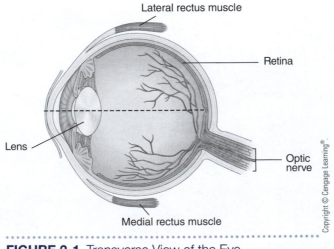

FIGURE 2-1 Transverse View of the Eye

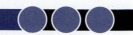

TASK 2-1B: MULTIPLE-CHOICE EXERCISE

Instructions: Circle the letter corresponding to the best answer to each of the following questions.

1. Ophthalmoscopy is also known as
   - A. endoscopy.
   - B. laryngoscopy.
   - C. fluoroscopy.
   - D. funduscopy.

2. A Snellen chart is used to measure
   - A. glaucoma pressure.
   - B. eye diameters.
   - C. visual acuity.
   - D. corneal reflexes.

3. The *white of the eye* is also known as the
   - A. choroid.
   - B. sclera.
   - C. conjunctiva.
   - D. iris.

4. A radial keratotomy is performed to treat
   - A. strabismus.
   - B. myopia.
   - C. cataracts.
   - D. hyperopia.

5. The condition in which the pupils are unequal in size is called
   - A. presbyopia.
   - B. astigmatism.
   - C. diplopia.
   - D. anisocoria.

6. The _____ is also known as the *blind spot* of the eye.
   - A. fovea centralis
   - B. optic disc
   - C. retina
   - D. optic nerve

7. The turning inward of the edge of the eyelid is called
   - A. entropion.
   - B. ectropion.
   - C. canthitis.
   - D. amblyopia.

8. Rods and cones are part of the anatomy of the
   - A. iris.
   - B. pupil.
   - C. retina.
   - D. macula.

9. The term _____ means *pertaining to the eye.*
   - A. ocular
   - B. extraocular
   - C. chorioid
   - D. lacrimal

10. Xerophthalmia is another name for
    A. nearsightedness.
    B. farsightedness.
    C. crossed eyes.
    D. dry eye.

TASK 2-1C: SPELLING CHOICE EXERCISE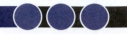

Instructions: Choose the correct spelling of each term.

1. fluorescein	floricine	fluroescine
2. capsulorehxis	capsulorrhexis	capsolorrhexis
3. myopia	miopia	meiopia
4. scitoma	skotoma	scotoma
5. mackula	maqula	macula
6. lacrimal	lacrimle	lacrimil
7. photcoagulation	photocoagulation	photocoglation
8. eridotomy	iridotomy	irridotomy
9. tonometry	tenometry	tonomitry
10. pupilary	puppilary	pupillary

TASK 2-2:   PROOFREADING EXERCISES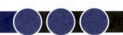

Instructions: The proofreading documents below are designed to challenge your proofreading and editing skills. The documents may contain missing demographic information, incorrect headings, misspelled words, misplaced punctuation, and other errors within the document. Read each report below and identify the error by circling the word. Then retype the document with the corrected text and formatting. When finished, proofread your work and save the document to your student disk using a different file name.

PROOFREADING EXERCISE 1

PREOPERATIVE DIAGNOSE: Senile cataract, right eye.

POSTOPERATIVE DIAGNOSIS: Senile cataract, right eye.

SURGEON(S): John J. Smith, MD

OPERATION: Phaco emulsification with posterior chamber intraocular lens, right eye.

INDICATIONS: Decreased vision, right eye.

procedure, the patient received several sets of drops into the right eye including 2-1/25% phenylephrine, 1% mydriacyl, Ocuflox, and Oculer. She was then taken to the operating room and sedated via I.V. sedation. Retrobulbar anesthesia was performed using a 50/50 mixture of 2% lidocaine and 0.75 percent Marcaine. The right eye was prepped using a 10% betadine solution. She was covered in a sterile drape, leaving only the right eye exposed.

(Continues)

PROOFREADING EXERCISE 1 *(Continued)*

A lid speculum was placed to provide exposure. A fixation ring and a super blade were used to create a pericentesis at approximately the 2:00 position. Viscoat was then injected through the paracentesis to fill the anterior chamber with the Thornton fixation ring, a 2.75 mm keratome blade was then used to create a two-step full-thickness clear corneal incision superiorly. The cystitome and Utrata forceps were then used to create a continuous capsulorhexes in the anterior lens capsule. bss on a hydrodissection cannula was used to perform gentle hydrodissection.

Phacoemulsification was then performed to remove the nuclear. Irrigation and aspiration were performed to remove the remaining cortical material. Provisc was then injected to fill the capsular bag and the anterior chamber. The intraocular lens was then injected into the capsular bag. The Kuglen hook was used to rotate the lens into proper position in the capsular bag. Irrigation and aspiration were then performed to remove the remaining viscal elastic material from the eye. BSS on a 30-gauge cannula was then used to hydrated the wound. The wounds were checked and found to be watertight. Lid speculum and drapes were carefully removed, several drops of Ocuflox were placed in the left eye followed by Maxitrol ointment. The eye was covered with a patch and shield. The patient was taken to the recovery area in good condition. There were no complications.

PROOFREADING EXERCISE 2

PREOPERATIVE DIAGNOSIS: Glacoma, uncontrolled intraocular pressure, right eye.

POSTOPERATIVE DIAGNOSIS: Glacoma, uncontrolled intraocular pressure, right eye.

SURGEON(S): John J. Smith, MD

OPERATION: Trabeculectomy with 5-FU, right eye.

PROCEDURE: After the risks and benefits of glaucoma surgery were discussed with the patient and his wife, legal guardian, informed consent was obtained. On the day of surgery, patient received several sets of drops including Zymar in the right eye. He was then taken to the operating room and sedated with IV sedation by anesthesia service. Retrobulbar anesthesia was given in the right eye. The right eye was prepped and draped in sterile fashion. Lid speculum was then placed to provide good exposure. A 40 silk was then used for superior rectus traction suture. The eye was then rotated down to provide good exposure superonasally.

Smooth forceps and westcott scissors were then used to create a peritomy about 8 to 9 mm from the limbis. The conjunctiva was then dissected down to bare sclera to create a limbal-based conjunctival flap. Area was cauterized with the eraser-tip cautery. Sponges soaked in 5-FU were then placed underneath the subconjunctival space and it was allowed to sit for 4 minutes checked against the clock. Sponges was then removed. The area was then irrigated with BSS. A razor blade on a blade breaker was then used to outline the trapezoid-shaped scleral flap and the flap was then dissected down to clear cornea with #64 blade. The 0.12 was used to lift the scleral flap and than the anterior chamber was then entered underneath the scleral flap with the sickle blade. A block of limbal tissue was then removed with the Kelly punch.

(Continues)

PROOFREADING EXERCISE 2 *(Continued)*

Iridectomy was then performed. BSS was then irrigated to reposition the iris back and the surgical iridectomy was then visible through clear cornua. Scleral flap was then repositioned and closed with the 10-0 Nylon on releasable suture fashion. The conjunctival flap was then closed with the 8-0 vicryl on BV needles. The traction suture was then removed. The lid speculum and drape were removed. Zymar was then placed. Maxitrol ointment was in place in the right eye. The right eye was pached with the eye patch and covered with the eye shield. The patient tolerated the procedure well. There were no complications.

 # OPHTHALMOLOGY TRANSCRIPTION **TIPS**

1. Watch for the soundalike words *macula, macule,* and *macular.* The *macula* is a small area located on the retina in the back of the eye. A *macule* is a small, flat, pigmented spot on the skin. *Macular,* an adjective, can refer to either the macula of the eye or a macule on the skin.

2. The notation of visual acuity is transcribed as a fraction, with normal vision written as 20/20 (dictated as "twenty twenty" or "twenty over twenty"). The first number will always be 20, indicating the 20 feet between the chart and the patient, and the second number will indicate a score attributed to a script the patient reads. For example, for a patient who reads the script at the score of 60 at 20 feet, the visual acuity is written as 20/60. A dictated value that sounds like a first number that is larger than 20, such as "twenty two hundred," would be transcribed as 20/200, not 2200 or 22/100.

3. The abbreviations *OD, OS,* and *OU,* which are often heard in the dictation of ophthalmology reports, stand for *oculus dexter* (right eye), *oculus sinister* (left eye), and *oculus uterque* (both eyes). These abbreviations should be expanded in the general text of the report. However, it is appropriate, and may even be preferred, to use the abbreviated forms when the text is associated with visual testing and measured values, unless instructed otherwise by your employer.

4. Remember to distinguish between the singular or plural form of the terms *sclera* and *conjunctiva* when transcribing dictation about these anatomical structures. When referring to both eyes, the plural forms of these terms are *sclerae* and *conjunctivae.*

5. In ophthalmology reports, physicians may refer to *forced duction,* which is a manual maneuver done to conduct passive movement of the eyeball in a particular direction. Do not mistranscribe this term as *forced adduction.*

TASK 2-3: CLOZE EXERCISES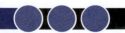

Instructions: The audio files for the following cloze exercises are located on the Premium website that accompanies this text (ISBN-13: 978-1-285-73537-5) at http://www.CengageBrain.com. If this is the first time you are registering your account, see the Preface for further instructions.

Once you are logged in to your account, locate the dictation file and Word document for the following cloze exercises. Open the audio file to be reviewed according to the exercise number indicated, along with its corresponding Word document. Listen to the dictation and read along with the text, filling in the missing words in the report by thinking critically and analytically about the context of the text you are reading. When finished, proofread your work and save the document according to your instructor's directions.

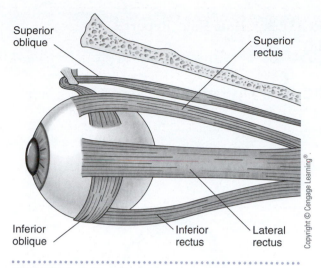

Superior oblique

Superior rectus

Inferior oblique

Inferior rectus

Lateral rectus

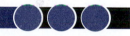

FIGURE 2-2 The Muscles of the Eye

CLOZE EXERCISE 1: Clinic Note_Report 6
Patient Name: Pamela Woods
Medical Record Number: 91921

CLOZE EXERCISE 2: Clinic Note_Report 7
Patient Name: Jun Lee
Medical Record Number: 32047

TASK 2-4: TRANSCRIPTION EXERCISES

Instructions: The audio files for the following transcription exercises are located on the Premium website that accompanies this text (ISBN-13: 978-1-285-73537-5) at http://www.CengageBrain.com. If this is the first time you are registering your account, see the Preface for further instructions.

Once you are logged in to your account, locate and open the audio file to be transcribed according to the exercise number indicated and transcribe each report. Do not insert a heading into the document if the text requires a second page, but let the text wrap naturally to the second page and continue typing. Transcribe the reports using the formatting specifics indicated in the Document Formatting Guidelines located at the beginning of this book. When finished, proofread your work and save the document according to your instructor's directions.

TRANSCRIPTION EXERCISE 1: Clinic Note_Report 16
Patient Name: Amanda Tucker
Medical Record Number: 86377

TRANSCRIPTION EXERCISE 2: Clinic Note_Report 1
Patient Name: Alice Freeman
Medical Record Number: 95093

TRANSCRIPTION EXERCISE 3: **Clinic Note_Report 2**
Patient Name: Steven Wright
Medical Record Number: 22530

TRANSCRIPTION EXERCISE 4: **Operative Note_Report 1**
Patient Name: Austin Brown
Medical Record Number: 15929

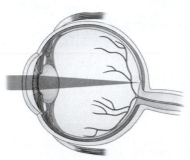

(A) Normal vision
Light rays focus on the retina.

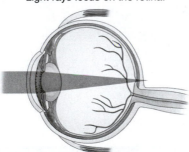

(B) Hyperopia (farsightedness)
Light rays focus beyond
the retina.

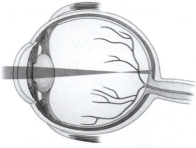

(C) Myopia (nearsightedness)
Light rays focus in front
of the retina.

Copyright © Cengage Learning®.

FIGURE 2-3 Refractive Disorders.
(A) Normal Vision. (B) Hyperopia.
(C) Myopia

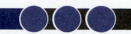

TASK 2-5 SPEECH RECOGNITION EXERCISES

Instructions: The audio files for the following speech recognition exercises are located on the Premium website that accompanies this text (ISBN-13: 978-1-285-73537-5) at http://www.CengageBrain.com. If this is the first time you are registering your account, see the Preface for further instructions.

Once you are logged in to your account, locate the dictation file and Word document for the following speech recognition exercises. Open the audio file to be reviewed according to the exercise number indicated, along with its corresponding Word document. Listen to the dictation and read along with the text, making corrections to the text with regard to formatting, terminology, grammar, spelling, and punctuation. When finished, proofread your work and save the document according to your instructor's directions.

SRT EXERCISE 1: Operative Report_Report S-20

Patient Name: Mario Bozzi

Medical Record Number: 08783

SRT EXERCISE 2: Operative Report_Report 6

Patient Name: Jean Porter

Medical Record Number: 57169

COMPUTER SOFTWARE **TIPS**

1. Use **AutoCorrect** to insert text used repetitively in medical reports. Click the **Microsoft Office** button located in the upper left corner of the Word document screen, then **Word Options** at the bottom of the window. Click **Proofing**. Click **AutoCorrect Options**. In the **Replace** box, type a word or phrase that you often mistype or misspell. In the **With** box, type the correct spelling of the word. Then click **Add**.

2. Word's spell check program allows you to add words to a custom dictionary. You can back up your custom dictionary by searching in Windows for any file with a **.doc** file extension. You can then copy those files to a memory stick or other storage media.

3. You can instruct Word to automatically save your work periodically. Choose the **Microsoft Office** button located in the upper left corner of the Word document screen. Select **Word Options** at the bottom of the window, then **Save** from the list on the left side of the **Word Options** box. On the right side of the window, check the box next to **Save Autorecover Information Every X Minutes**. You can change the value in the drop-down box to a value you feel comfortable with. Click OK to close the window.

4. Use the CTRL key to move quickly around a document. Press **CTRL + HOME** to move to the top of the document. To move to the bottom of a document, press **CTRL + END**. To go to the top of the next page, press **CTRL + PAGE DOWN** and to move to the top of the preceding page, press **CTRL + PAGE UP**.

5. To select a word, simply double-click on it. If a space immediate follows the word you select, the space gets selected, too. Punctuation is ignored.

OPHTHALMOLOGY BOOK OF STYLE **TIPS**

1. The term *adnexa oculi* refers to the accessory organs of the eye: the eyelids, lashes, brows, lacrimal apparatus, and extrinsic muscles of the eyeball. Note this term is always written in plural, even if the dictating physician is talking about only one eye. Be sure to follow this term with a plural verb.

2. Lasers are used often in ophthalmologic surgery and should be transcribed as dictated. Be sure to check a reliable medical dictionary or other resource for the exact brand name spelling of these tools. Some common lasers used include:

   argon laser

   Victus Femtosecond Laser Platform

   YAG laser

   holmium: YAG laser

3. The term *cup-to-disc ratio* refers to the ratio of the diameter of the optic cup to the diameter of the optic disc, and should always be hyphenated.

4. When describing the optic status of the patient, physicians will dictate a positive or negative number (dictating the words "plus" or "minus") with decimal values. Transcribe these values with a positive or negative sign with no space between the symbol and the decimal value. For example:

   Dictated: It was found that the patient has a plus twelve lens.

   Transcribed: It was found that the patient had a +12.00 lens.

5. Do not use the word "disk" in ophthalmologic references. You should use *disc* for all references to the optic disc in ophthalmology. The word *disk* is used for all anatomical terms other than ophthalmologic use, including the disks of the spine.

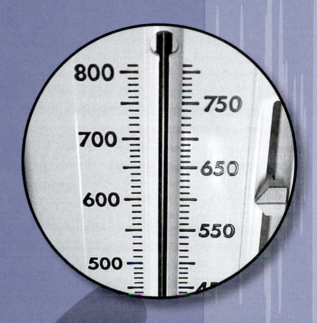

PROJECT 3

Pulmonology

TASK 3-1A: SOUNDALIKE TERM REVIEW EXERCISE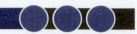

Instructions: Circle the correct pulmonary term in the following sentences.

1. Lung sounds that resemble crackles indicating that the lung is partly filled with fluid are called (**rales, rails**).

2. After obtaining a positive tuberculin skin test, I informed the patient that she likely had (**TB, TV**) and would need treatment right away.

3. Doctors typically use Lasix to decrease the pressure in the lungs caused by pulmonary (**erythema, edema**).

4. The patient's (**bronchoscopy, rhinoscopy**) showed moderate tracheitis and no masses.

5. His pulmonary function tests showed an (**FBV1, FEV1**) of 3.2L.

6. The trachea branches off into two main (**bronchi, rhonchi**).

7. The actual exchange of gases in the lungs occurs at the (**areoli, alveoli**).

8. The patient's recent CT scan showed a (**pleural, plural**) effusion in the right lower lobe.

9. Her lung exam showed (**course, coarse**) rhonchi throughout.

10. The reason for the patient's visit was (**pruritic, pleuritic**) chest pain since last night.

11. The patient recently underwent a ventilation (**profusion, perfusion**) scan, which was normal.

12. Enlargement of the right ventricle of the heart in response to increased resistance or high blood pressure in the lungs is called (**corp, cor**) pulmonale.

13. (**Arthrosis, Anthracosis**) is a lung condition resulting from long-term exposure to coal dust.

14. The presence of air in the lungs, called (**pneumothorax, hemothorax**), is generally diagnosed by chest x-ray.

15. In the chest, the trachea divides into the right and left main (**bronchiole, bronchus**).

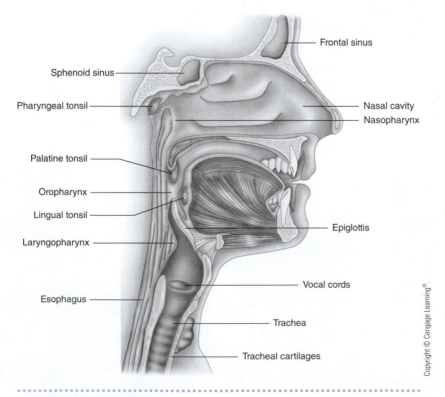

FIGURE 3-1 Structures of the Upper Respiratory Tract

TASK 3-1B: FILL IN THE BLANKS EXERCISE

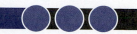

Instructions: Write the correct answer on the line provided.

1. A barrel chest is often seen in patients with _____.

2. The surgeon removed a portion of the patient's lung. This procedure is known as a _____.

3. The baby was not receiving enough oxygen, causing his skin to appear blue. The medical term for *bluish condition* is _____.

4. The elderly patient inhaled food into his lung while eating, which caused _____ pneumonia.

5. The patient suffered from respiratory failure and a _____ was performed, which consisted of creating a stoma into the trachea to insert a temporary tube to facilitate breathing.

6. The child was hit in the nose with a ball, causing her nose to bleed, a condition known as _____.

7. The medical term for a *sore throat* is _____.

8. The two large tubes that branch out from the trachea to convey air into the two lungs are called the _____.

9. The patient's wife noted that his breathing would repeatedly stop and start during sleep, a condition called _____.

10. The surgical removal of the larynx is called a _____.

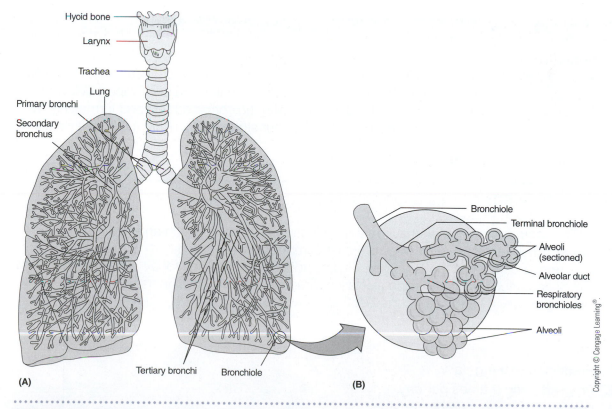

FIGURE 3-2 The Right and Left Lung Anatomy. (A) The Trachea and Bronchial Tree. (B) The Bronchioles, Alveolar Duct, and Alveoli

TASK 3-1C: ABBREVIATIONS EXERCISE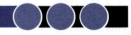

Instructions: Write the expansion of each abbreviation.

1. MRI   _____

2. COPD   _____

3. CPAP   _____

4. BAL   _____

5. PE   _____

6. TB   _____

7. ABG   _____

8. DVT   _____

9. CPR   _____

10. CXR   _____

11. ARDS   _____

12. RF   _____

13. ETT   _____

14. URI   _____

15. PFT   _____

TASK 3-2:   PROOFREADING EXERCISES

Instructions: The proofreading documents below are designed to challenge your proofreading and editing skills. The documents may contain missing demographic information, incorrect headings, misspelled words, misplaced punctuation, and other errors within the document. Read each report below and identify the error by circling the word. Then retype the document with the corrected text and formatting. When finished, proofread your work and save the document to your student disk using a different file name.

PROOFREADING EXERCISE 1

REASON FOR VISIT: Lung transplant follow up.

HISTORY: As an outpatient, we have been monitoring his renal function and noticed a progressive rise in his creatine over the past 2 months, most recently 4-1/2 as of yesterday from a baseline in the 2.5 range. He has additional complains today of cough and mild clear sputum production and also a low-grade fever. Moreover, he has nausea and vomiting as well as diarrhea for the last 2 to 3 days.

MEDICATIONS:

1. Prednisone 10 mg daily.
2. Prograft 5 mg 2 times per day.
3. Dapsone 100 mg 3 times per week.

(Continues)

PROOFREADING EXERCISE 1 *(Continued)*

4. Prevacid 30 mg daily.
5. Aranesp 100 mg every week.
6. Flonase 4 puffs 2 times per day.
7. Atrovent as needed.

FINDINGS: Temperature 99.5, pulse 100, blood pressure 112/81, and pulse oximetry on room air is 96%. His lungs have occasional ronchi at the right bases. The remainder of the physical exam is unremarkable.

ASSESSMENT: Status post bilateral lung transplants for sarcoidosis with multiple issues, including significant fall in pulmonary function, low grade fever, worsening azotemia, and anemia, rule out hemolytis.

PLAN: We will admit this patient and puruse the following:

1. Intervenous hydration.
2. Radiographic assessment of his lung and bronchoscopy in the morning.
3. Renal consultation. If there is no reversible cause, we may consider discontinuing the calciurin inhibitor and substituting rapamycin.
4. We will work him up for hemolysis and stop the Dapsone.

PROOFREADING EXERCISE 2

DIAGNOSIS:

1. Bronchitis.
2. Chronic obstruction pulmonary disease.

PROCEDURES PERFORMED: Chest X-ray showed increased markings in left lower lung, possibly early left lower lobe pneumonia versus chronic fibrosis, minimal hyperinflation with flattened diaphragms, decreased lung markings, both upper lungs, and increased AP diameter. Chest compatible with emphysema. Moderate diffuse osteoporosis. Wedging one midthoracic vertebral body.

CHIEF COMPLAINT: Cough with white frothy sputum, with shortness of breath and dispnea on exertion, worse for 3 days.

HISTORY OF PRESENT ILLNESS: This is an 83-year-old african american male with COPD and diagnosed with a non-ST-elevation MI at the VA Hospital in Baltimore, Maryland 1 one half months ago. Patient underwent cardiac catheterization at that time and was discharged on Plavix. The patient says that many prescription changes were made as well. The patient reports ongoing dyspnea on exertion and shortness of breath since then. Most recently the patent complained of very severe cough with white sputum. No hemoptysis. The patient denies chest pain. He does have nocturnia and PND, subjective hot and cold flashes but denies night sweats or weightloss.

(Continues)

PROOFREADING EXERCISE 2 *(Continued)*

HOSPITAL COURSE: I believe the patient has sever COPD, but the patient does not want to have PFT's done because he does not want to pay the expense since he can get them done for free at the VA. The patient also does not want to have act to make sure he does not have a PE, although my previous probability for a PE was low. The patient also refuses to be transferred to the VA where he can receive these studies for free. The patient decided he would rather be discharged. The patient was treated for bronchitis with doxicycline.

On the day of discharge the patient's vital signs were good. Patient was afebrile, heart rate 87, blood pressure 108/62, respiratory rate 18. His saturation was 95% on 2 liters or 94% on room air. He desaturated to 89% while ambulating.

DISCHARGE MEDICATIONS: Please restart home medications except to increase Toprol XR from 25 mg to 50 mg daily. Prescription was given.

DISCHARGE INSTRUCTIONS:

1. Diet: Cardiac diet.
2. Activity: The patient was told to go to the VA Hospital to set up home physical therapy and pulmonary rehab. No activity restrictions but he should walk with assistance. He should continue to be active.

FOLLOWUP INSTRUCTIONS: The patient was told to call his doctor for worsening shortness of breath, chest pane, vomiting, or any new or worrisome systems. The patient will see his doctor in the VA Hospital in the next 1 to 2 weeks. Please call the VA Hospital to set up home physical therapy and pulmonary rehabiltation.

PULMONOLOGY TRANSCRIPTION **TIPS**

1. A *Pleur-evac*, which is a water-seal suction device for pulmonary procedures, is correctly transcribed with a capital "P" only and the hyphen, not "Pleurovac."

2. Watch for these pulmonology-related soundalike words:
   - *pleural*: Relating to the delicate serous membrane that lines each half of the thorax.
   - *plural*: Relating to more than one kind.
   - *pleuritic*: Relating to pleurisy, an inflammation of the pleura of the chest.
   - *pruritic*: Pertaining to pruritus, or itching.
   - *perfusion*: Relating to the amount of blood reaching a tissue.
   - *profusion*: Relating to something that is present in abundance.
   - *bronchi*: Pleural of *bronchus*, one of the two subdivisions of the trachea serving to convey air to and from the lungs.
   - *rhonchi*: An added sound with a musical pitch occurring during inspiration or expiration, heard while listening to the chest during a physical exam.

3. The word *airway* can also be dictated in the plural, *airways*.

4. Physicians will often dictate the words *tracheostomy* and *tracheotomy* as "trach" interchangeably, as these words are synonymous. Therefore, unless you know for sure which term the dictator is referring to, you should not expand this word.

5. Spell out "breaths per minute" and "respirations per minute." Do not abbreviate as *bpm* or *rpm*, respectively.

TASK 3-3: CLOZE EXERCISES
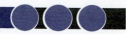

Instructions: The audio files for the following cloze exercises are located on the Premium website that accompanies this text (ISBN-13: 978-1-285-73537-5) at http://www.CengageBrain.com. If this is the first time you are registering your account, see the Preface for further instructions.

Once you are logged in to your account, locate the dictation file and Word document for the following cloze exercises. Open the audio file to be reviewed according to the exercise number indicated, along with its corresponding Word document. Listen to the dictation and read along with the text, filling in the missing words in the report by thinking critically and analytically about the context of the text you are reading. When finished, proofread your work and save the document according to your instructor's directions.

CLOZE EXERCISE 1: Chest X-ray_Report 3341
Patient Name: Aizah Sharma
Medical Record Number: 57425

CLOZE EXERCISE 2: Clinic Note_Report 11
Patient Name: Donald Scott
Medical Record Number: 10241

TASK 3-4: TRANSCRIPTION EXERCISES
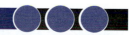

Instructions: The audio files for the following transcription exercises are located on the Premium website that accompanies this text (ISBN-13: 978-1-285-73537-5) at http://www.CengageBrain.com. If this is the first time you are registering your account, see the Preface for further instructions.

Once you are logged in to your account, locate and open the audio file to be transcribed according to the exercise number indicated and transcribe each report. Do not insert a heading into the document if the text requires a second page, but let the text wrap naturally to the second page and continue typing. Transcribe the reports using the formatting specifics indicated in the Document Formatting Guidelines located at the beginning of this book. When finished, proofread your work and save the document according to your instructor's directions.

TRANSCRIPTION EXERCISE 1: Clinic Note_Report 9001
Patient Name: Edmund White
Medical Record Number: 26503

TRANSCRIPTION EXERCISE 2: Discharge Summary_Report 5
Patient Name: Angela Garza
Medical Record Number: 50424

TRANSCRIPTION EXERCISE 3: Clinic Note_Report 4
Patient Name: Neil Anderson
Medical Record Number: 04954

TRANSCRIPTION EXERCISE 4: Clinic Note_Report 5
Patient Name: Matthew Thompson
Medical Record Number: 42365

TRANSCRIPTION EXERCISE 5: Clinic Note_Report 2
Patient Name: Rebecca McDonald
Medical Record Number: 02839

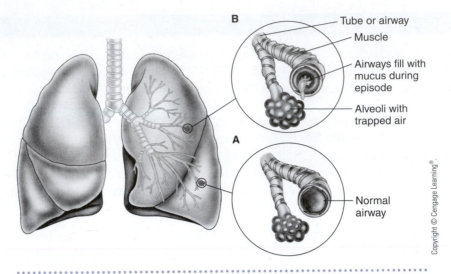

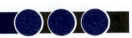

FIGURE 3-3 Asthma. (A) Before the Episode, the Muscles are Relaxed and the Airways are Open. (B) During the Episode, the Muscles Tighten and the Airways Fill with Mucus.

TASK 3-5: SPEECH RECOGNITION EXERCISES

Instructions: The audio files for the following speech recognition exercises are located on the Premium website that accompanies this text (ISBN-13: 978-1-285-73537-5) at http://www.CengageBrain.com. If this is the first time you are registering your account, see the Preface for further instructions.

Once you are logged in to your account, locate the dictation file and Word document for the following speech recognition exercises. Open the audio file to be reviewed according to the exercise number indicated, along with its corresponding Word document. Listen to the dictation and read along with the text, making corrections to the text with regard to formatting, terminology, grammar, spelling, and punctuation. When finished, proofread your work and save the document according to your instructor's directions.

SRT EXERCISE 1: **Emergency Room Note_Report 9**
Patient Name: Joseph Long
Medical Record Number: 48709

SRT EXERCISE 2: **CT Scan of the Chest_Report 3213**
Patient Name: Hidi Kalu
Medical Record Number: 82804

SRT EXERCISE 3: **Discharge Summary_Report 2**
Patient Name: George Leon
Medical Record Number: 99231

SRT EXERCISE 4: **Discharge Summary_Report 3**
Patient Name: Cassandra Hunter
Medical Record Number: 33018

COMPUTER SOFTWARE **TIPS**

1. To quickly change line spacing in a document, highlight the selected text and press **CTRL + 1** for single spacing or **CTRL + 2** for double spacing.

2. Use the F4 key to repeat a last action.

3. A fast way to locate a synonym for a word is to select the word and right-click it. In the menu, select **synonyms** and click your desired replacement.

4. MicroSoft Word allows you to select text quickly using the mouse.
   - To select a word, double-click the word using the left mouse button.
   - To select a sentence, press and hold CTRL and single-click on the sentence using the left mouse button.
   - To select a line of text on the screen, single-click in the left screen margin at the line you want to select with the left mouse button.
   - To select a paragraph, triple-click in the paragraphs using the left mouse button.
   - To select the whole document, press and hold **CTRL + A**, or triple-click in the left margin of the screen using the left mouse button.

5. You can automatically keep dates current in your documents. Choose **Insert**, then choose **Date and Time**, and then select the date format you want for the document. Then check the small box at the bottom next to **Update Automatically**.

PULMONOLOGY BOOK OF STYLE **TIPS**

1. When transcribing gas abbreviations, use uppercase letters and subscripts, or place the numerals on the same line. Make sure you do not type the zero key, for the capital "O" key. "O" in these abbreviations stands for "oxygen."

   $CO2$ or CO_2

   $O2$ or O_2

   The letters may be combined with numbers in capital or lowercase letters when used in pulmonary function testing and other respiratory physiology.

   $PO2$, PO_2 or $pO2$, pO_2

   $PCO2$, PCO_2 or $pCO2$, pCO_2

   $PaO2$ or PaO_2

   $PaCO2$ or $PaCO_2$

2. The following abbreviations are commonly used in reference to mechanical ventilation and airway management. Unless instructed to the contrary by your employer, you may use these abbreviations without expanding them first in a document.

BiPAP	bilevel positive airway pressure
CPAP	continuous positive airway pressure
ET	endotracheal tube
NIPPV	noninvasive positive pressure ventilation
PEEP	positive end-expiratory pressure

3. When transcribing the phrase "liters of oxygen," do not insert a space between the numeric value and the unit of measure.

   The patient was placed on high-flow oxygen at a rate of 5L/min.

   The patient's oxygen saturation was 98% on 2L via nasal cannula.

4. Physicians use the Epworth Sleepiness Scale to measure daytime sleepiness in a patient when assessing a potential sleep disorder. The scale measures from 1 to 24 and values are assigned to different scenarios by the patient, such as when sitting and reading or watching television. Transcribe this score using initial capital letters along with the numeric value.

The patient's Epworth Sleepiness Scale score was calculated to be 18.

5. There are many abbreviations associated with pulmonary function tests (PFTs). These abbreviations should be transcribed using all capital letters with numerals on the same line, unless instructed otherwise. The following of these abbreviations are the most common in medical reports:

FEF	forced expiratory flow
FEV	forced expiratory volume
FEV1 (or FEV$_1$)	FEV in first second of expiration
FIO2 (or FIO$_2$)	fraction of inspired oxygen
FVC	forced vital capacity
TLC	total lung capacity
DLCO	carbon monoxide diffusing capacity
TV	tidal volume

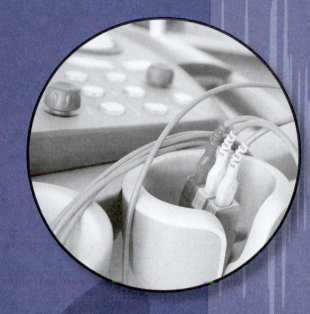

PROJECT 4

Cardiology

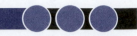

Instructions: Read the clinic note below and answer the questions that follow by choosing the correct letter answer.

CLINIC NOTE

Ms. Anna Calantini comes to the cardiology clinic accompanied by her daughter who provides translation services. She is a 52-year-old Hispanic female referred to us from Endocrinology for "preventive cardiac testing and lower extremity edema."

The patient does not have any history of established heart disease of any sort. Her coronary risk factors include diabetes of 5 years' duration, hypertension of 9 years' duration, treated hyperlipidemia, and a positive family history in that a brother had a bypass surgery at approximately the age of 60. She has never been a tobacco user. Her primary doctor is a Dr. Garcia who has been managing her blood pressure and her lipids.

The patient leads a very sedentary existence with physical activity largely limited to minimum activity within the house and occasionally ambulating somewhat outside the house. She never experiences any chest discomfort or dyspnea with this. She does have occasional nocturnal dyspnea that she attributes to bronchospasm, which responds to the use of a bronchodilator.

On physical examination, she is an obese female with no acute distress. Her weight is 240 pounds, height 5 feet 2 inches, blood pressure 144/82, and pulse 100 and regular. Her lungs were clear to auscultation. On neck examination, her jugular venous pulse was somewhat difficult to assess because of the width of her neck; however, it appeared to be less than 5 cms with no hepatojugular reflex. Her carotid upstrokes were normal bilaterally with no bruits. Her cardiac exam revealed normal S1 and S2 with no murmurs or gallops. Her ankles had 1+ bilateral edema with intact pedal pulses.

Her electrocardiogram today was normal.

Her lipids today revealed an LDL of 4 and HDL of 40.

ASSESSMENT AND PLAN

1. Ankle edema. I suspect that her dependent edema is largely due to some mild venous insufficiency and more likely related to her obesity interfering with good venous return. I do not detect any evidence of heart failure on exam. However, to fully address this issue, we will check a BNP and check an echocardiogram to assess her LV function.

2. Lipids. Her LDL is certainly at goal for someone with diabetes and I will not make any changes to her Lipitor.

3. Blood pressure. Her blood pressure today is not ideally controlled, but it is largely being managed by her primary care physician, so I will not make any adjustments today.

I will see her back when her echocardiogram is done, to review those results with her, but I am doubtful that we will identify any active cardiovascular issues at this time.

1. Ankle edema can be a cardiac symptom of
   A. an irregular heartbeat.
   B. heart failure.
   C. an impending heart attack.
   D. none of the above.

2. The physician would like to perform an echocardiogram in order to
   A. assess the potassium level of the heart.
   B. assess the electrical activity of the heart.
   C. assess the ventricular function of the heart.
   D. assess the chemical makeup of the heart.

3. The patient had good blood flow from the neck veins up to the brain. This is evident by the statement:
   A. "Her cardiac exam revealed normal S1 and S2."
   B. "Her lungs were clear to auscultation."
   C. "Her ankles had 1+ bilateral edema with intact pedal pulses."
   D. "Her carotid upstrokes were normal bilaterally with no bruits."

4. What term in the report indicates that the patient has high levels of cholesterol?
   A. Hypertension
   B. Hyperlipidemia
   C. Dyspnea
   D. Pedal edema

5. According to the physician, the patient's mild venous insufficiency is probably related to
   A. obesity.
   B. heart failure.
   C. an abnormal LDL.
   D. an abnormal echocardiogram result.

6. The patient attributes her nocturnal dyspnea to
   A. a sedentary lifestyle.
   B. her diabetes.
   C. bronchospasm.
   D. her 1+ pitting edema.

7. What is not included as a cardiac risk in this patient?
   A. Hypertension
   B. Tobacco smoking
   C. Hyperlipidemia
   D. Her height

8. What is the meaning of the word *sedentary*?
   A. Euphoric
   B. Active
   C. Out of balance
   D. Inactive

9. The phrase "S1 and S2" refers to
   A. heart sounds.
   B. respirations.
   C. murmurs.
   D. gallops.

10. Where is the jugular venous pulse located?
    A. In the legs
    B. In the forearms
    C. In the neck
    D. In the thigh

TASK 4-1B: COMBINING FORMS EXERCISE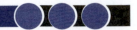

Instructions: Write the meaning of the cardiac combining form given.

1. arteri/o _____

2. ather/o _____

3. thromb/o _____

4. my/o _____

5. palpit/o _____

6. ectop/o _____

7. cardi/o _____

8. isch/o _____

9. cyan/o _____

10. valv/o _____

11. sten/o _____

12. atri/o _____

13. vascul/o _____

14. ven/o _____

15. angi/o _____

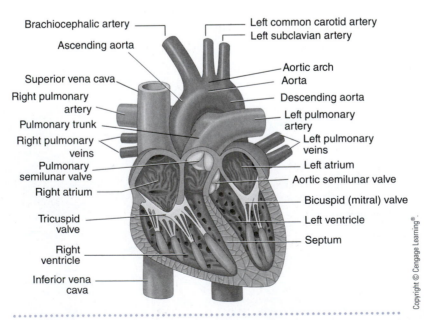

FIGURE 4-1 Internal View of the Heart, its Chambers, Valves, and Great Vessels

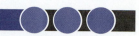

TASK 4-1C: FILL IN THE BLANKS EXERCISE

Instructions: Fill in the name of the lab test with the description of the test given. Each test name can be used more than once.

oximetry   cardiac enzymes   lipid panel
BNP   sphygmomanometry
C-reactive protein   electrolyte panel

1. Blood pressure test _____

2. Found in blood when inflammation occurs _____

3. Na, K, Cl, and CO2 _____

4. Cholesterol, HDL, and LDL _____

5. Oxygen saturation of hemoglobin _____

6. Troponin, CK, and CPK _____

7. A hormone made by the heart _____

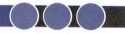

TASK 4-2: PROOFREADING EXERCISES

Instructions: The proofreading documents below are designed to challenge your proofreading and editing skills. The documents may contain missing demographic information, incorrect headings, misspelled words, misplaced punctuation, and other errors within the document. Read each report below and identify the error by circling the word. Then retype the document with the corrected text and formatting. When finished, proofread your work and save the document to your student disk using a different file name.

PROOFREADING EXERCISE 1

PROGRESS NOTE:

The patient returns today for an unsceduled visit at the request of his private physician for chest discomfort.

The patient states that he has had a chest cold for the past week. While setting up for an art show, he developed some chest heaviness. He felt it was secondary to an upper respiratory tract infection, as the chest discomfort did get worse with coughing. His cough was productive of brown yellow sputum. He was seen by his private physician and placed on amoxicillin and prednisone. He has also complained that at night he feels like he is not getting enough air into his lungs and has awakened up to take some deep, sighing breaths. He denies any orthopnea or PMD. He denies palpations, syncope, or any episodes of recurrent afterial fibrillation that he can relate to. He occasionally does drink caffeinated drinks still and has gained approximately fifteen pounds.

MEDICATIONS:

1. Synthroid.
2. Altace 10 mg q.d.
3. Prednisone.
4. Amoxicillin.

(Continues)

PROOFREADING EXERCISE 1 *(Continued)*

PHYSICAL EXAMINATION: Alert oriented in no acute distress. Blood pressure is 130/78, heart rate 65. Neck reveals jugular venous pressure of approximately 14 mmhg. There are no brutes noted. Lungs reveal bibasilar rails. Heart: Regular rate and rhythm, without murmurs, gallops, or rubs. Abdomen is soft, nontender, without mass or organomegaly. Extremities are without edema.

LABORATORY: EKG: PR interval 0.18. QRS interval 0.06. Axis zero degrees. Sinus rhythm, rate of 65. Small inferior Q-waves of unknown significance. Nonspecific ST and T-wave abnormalities. Essentially unchanged.

IMPRESSION: Chest pain. This patient has somewhat atypical chest discomfort, which may be, in fact, related to his recent upper respiratory infection. Because of his multiple coronary risk factors of hypertension, hypercholesteremia, and new onset of chest discomfort, we will plan to do an exercise myoview stress test in the next week or so.

PROOFREADING EXERCISE 2

EXERCISE TREADMILL TEST

This is a 40 year old gentleman status post aortic valve replacement secondary to endocarditis who is undergoing exercise treadmill testing as part of an entrance to a cardiac rehabilitation program.

MEDICATIONS:

1. Metoprolol 50 mg bid.
2. Lanoxin .25 mg daily.
3. Zoloft 50 mg daily.
4. Aspirin.

PROTOCOL: Standard bruce protocol.

RESTING EKG: PR interval 0.16. QRS 0.06. Axis plus 90 degrees.

Interpretation: Sinus rhythm, rate of 76. Minor diffuse, nonspecific ST and T-wave abnormalities.

RESULTS: Patient exercised for nine minutes, achieving a maximal heart rate of 140, which was 78% of his maximal predicted heart rate. Patient achieved 10 METs of exercise.

BLOOD PRESSURE: Initial resting blood pressure 118/78 and rose to a peak of 155/60 at peek exercise, then decreased to 138/75 five minutes in the recovery phase. Double product 21700.

(Continues)

PROOFREADING EXERCISE 2 *(Continued)*

SYMPTOMS: Patient experienced leg fatigue while on the treadmill but denied any chest tightness complaints.

REASON FOR STOPPING: Leg fatig.

STRESS EKG: There were no ST or T-wave abnormalities suggestive of iscemia.

ARRHYTHMIAS: There were no PVCs, PAC's, supraventricular or ventricular tachycardia noted.

IMPRESSION:

1. Good exercise tolerant.
2. Negative for development of chest discomfort.
3. Electrocardiogram non-diagnostic, less than 85% of maximal predicted heart rate.
4. Normal blood pressure response.

 CARDIOLOGY TRANSCRIPTION **TIPS**

1. Patients in the emergency room or cardiac care unit are said to have an *acute myocardial infarction.* Be careful not to hear this incorrectly as "mild cardiac infarction."

2. A portion of a report that discusses the patient's cardiac status may include the term *cor*, referring to the heart. The soundalike word *core* refers to the central part of anything. Do not mistranscribe the word *cor* for the word *core.* *Cor* may also be dictated as a subheading in a physical exam.

3. When a patient tires easily, the word often dictated is *fatigability.* The "u" that appears in *fatigue* should be dropped from this other form of the word.

4. The third and fourth heart sounds (S3 and S4, respectively) are abnormal sounds caused by heart wall vibration. You will never hear "normal S3 and S4" in dictation but perhaps "*no* S3 or S4."

5. Plaques that form in the arteries are referred to as a condition known as *atherosclerosis*, not the soundalike word *arthrosclerosis*, which refers to stiffness of the joints, especially in the aged.

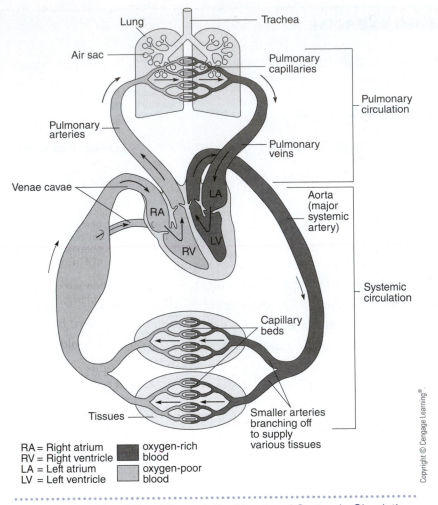

RA = Right atrium
RV = Right ventricle
LA = Left atrium
LV = Left ventricle

oxygen-rich blood
oxygen-poor blood

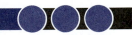

FIGURE 4-2 Blood Flow Through the Heart and Systemic Circulation

TASK 4-3: CLOZE EXERCISES

Instructions: The audio files for the following cloze exercises are located on the Premium website that accompanies this text (ISBN-13: 978-1-285-73537-5) at http://www.CengageBrain.com. If this is the first time you are registering your account, see the Preface for further instructions.

Once you are logged in to your account, locate the dictation file and Word document for the following cloze exercises. Open the audio file to be reviewed according to the exercise number indicated, along with its corresponding Word document. Listen to the dictation and read along with the text, filling in the missing words in the report by thinking critically and analytically about the context of the text you are reading. When finished, proofread your work and save the document according to your instructor's directions.

CLOZE EXERCISE 1: Progress Note_Report 7106
Patient Name: Edward West
Medical Record Number: 33104

CLOZE EXERCISE 2: Exercise Treadmill Test_Report 7154
Patient Name: Hamza Aziz
Medical Record Number: 83204

TASK 4-4: TRANSCRIPTION EXERCISES

Instructions: The audio files for the following transcription exercises are located on the Premium website that accompanies this text (ISBN-13: 978-1-285-73537-5) at http://www.CengageBrain.com. If this is the first time you are registering your account, see the Preface for further instructions.

Once you are logged in to your account, locate and open the audio file to be transcribed according to the exercise number indicated and transcribe each report. Do not insert a heading into the document if the text requires a second page, but let the text wrap naturally to the second page and continue typing. Transcribe the reports using the formatting specifics indicated in the Document Formatting Guidelines located at the beginning of this book. When finished, proofread your work and save the document according to your instructor's directions.

TRANSCRIPTION EXERCISE 1: Admission History and Physical_Report 7124
Patient Name: Janet Burns
Medical Record Number: 05611

TRANSCRIPTION EXERCISE 2: 2-D Echocardiogram_Report 7119
Patient Name: Alice Freeman
Medical Record Number: 92978

TRANSCRIPTION EXERCISE 3: 24-hour Holter Monitor _Report 7178
Patient Name: Alfredo Diaz
Medical Record Number: 28875

TRANSCRIPTION EXERCISE 4: Adenosine Thallium Stress Test_Report 7167
Patient Name: Sarah Silva
Medical Record Number: 95894

TRANSCRIPTION EXERCISE 5: Discharge Summary_Report 7196
Patient Name: Nancy Black
Medical Record Number: 40250

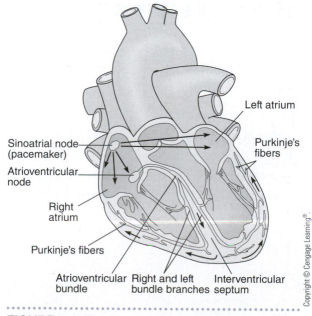

Left atrium

Purkinje's fibers

Sinoatrial node (pacemaker)

Atrioventricular node

Right atrium

Purkinje's fibers

Atrioventricular bundle

Right and left bundle branches

Interventricular septum

FIGURE 4-3 The Conduction System of the Heart

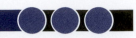

TASK 4-5: SPEECH RECOGNITION EXERCISES

Instructions: The audio files for the following speech recognition exercises are located on the Premium website that accompanies this text (ISBN-13: 978-1-285-73537-5) at http://www.CengageBrain.com. If this is the first time you are registering your account, see the Preface for further instructions.

Once you are logged in to your account, locate the dictation file and Word document for the following speech recognition exercises. Open the audio file to be reviewed according to the exercise number indicated, along with its corresponding Word document. Listen to the dictation and read along with the text, making corrections to the text with regard to formatting, terminology, grammar, spelling, and punctuation. When finished, proofread your work and save the document according to your instructor's directions.

SRT EXERCISE 1: Progress Note_Report 7102
Patient Name: Carol Cunningham
Medical Record Number: 09184

SRT EXERCISE 2: History and Physical Examination_Report 7168
Patient Name: Dorothy Mason
Medical Record Number: 29675

SRT EXERCISE 3: Progress Note_Report 7120
Patient Name: Dorothy Miller
Medical Record Number: 74400

SRT EXERCISE 4: 2-D Echocardiogram_Report 7172
Patient Name: Alton Richards III
Medical Record Number: 84511

COMPUTER SOFTWARE **TIPS**

1. To highlight all instances of specific text in a document, in the **Find** box, click **Reading Highlight,** then click **Highlight All**.

2. When using AutoCorrect, note that Word inserts the AutoCorrect entry in a document only when you press the spacebar after typing the text you want Word to correct. This prevents an AutoCorrect entry from being inserted inappropriately. For example, Word will insert "Robert Dawson" when you type "rd" followed by a space, but not when you type "Maple Rd."

3. By default, Word automatically creates a hyperlink to an e-mail address or the URL of a website when you type the address or URL in a document. To remove a hyperlink, right-click it, then click **Remove Hyperlink**. The hyperlink will be removed, but the text will remain in the document.

CARDIOLOGY BOOK OF STYLE **TIPS**

1. The abbreviations ECG and EKG are used interchangeably by physicians to describe an *electrocardiogram*, and both are acceptable. You may transcribe the abbreviations as dictated; however, many people in the medical field feel that for the sake of clarity in a medical document, *echocardiogram* and *electrocardiogram* should always be spelled out because ECG may also refer to either an electrocardiogram or an echocardiogram.

2. Murmurs are written using arabic numbers. Place a forward slash between the murmur grade and the scale used, even when the dictator may say "out of" or "over" to express these grades.

   Dictated: The patient had a grade 2 over 6 murmur.

   Transcribed: The patient had a grade 2/6 murmur.

   When a range is used to describe a murmur, break it out into two values.

   Dictated: The patient had a grade 4 to 5 over 6 murmur.

   Transcribed: The patient had a grade 4/6 to 5/6 murmur.

3. Dictators commonly dictate the ST segment and the T wave together, using the terms "ST wave" or "STT wave," but there is actually no such thing as an ST wave or an ST-T wave. These terms should be transcribed as follows:

Dictated	Transcribed
STT wave	ST and T wave
ST wave	ST segment and T wave

4. Do not use a hyphen for EKG tracing terms. However, do use the hyphen for EKG tracing terms when they are followed by and modifying a noun.

T wave	T-wave abnormality, ST and T-wave abnormality
ST segment	ST-segment depression
non-Q wave	non-Q-wave myocardial infarction

5. The New York Heart Association (NYHA) classification system is used to classify levels of heart failure. The classes are written in roman numerals.

   Dictated: The patient had a New York Heart Association class two cardiac failure.

   Transcribed: The patient had a New York Heart Association class II cardiac failure.

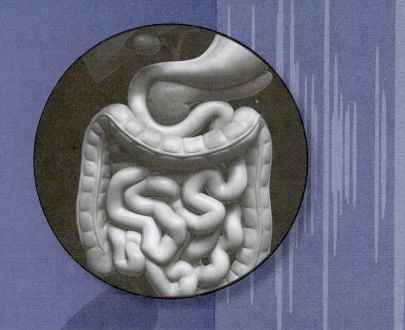

PROJECT 5

Gastroenterology

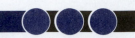

TASK 5-1A: FILL IN THE BLANKS EXERCISE

Instructions: Read the following clinic note and fill in the blanks in the record with the terms listed, relying on the context provided in the sentence to make your choices. Each term should be used only once.

syndrome	migraine	Oddi	MCV
cholecystectomy	pleuritic	quadrant	hepatitis
bowel	clubbing	pulposus	phosphatase
adhesions	percutaneous	cholelithiasis	atraumatic
anicteric	rhythm	CBC	blood

The patient presents with symptoms of abdominal pain. She underwent open _____ for symptomatic _____, and she was pain-free for approximately 15 years. The patient was subsequently diagnosed with chronic _____ C viral infection and underwent _____ liver biopsy approximately 2-1/2 years ago for pretreatment evaluation. Following the liver biopsy, the patient immediately developed severe right upper quadrant and right flank pain associated with _____ chest pain that lasted for approximately 1 week. Now she has developed recurrent attacks of right upper quadrant abdominal pain consistent with her previous biliary colic some 15 years prior. The patient denies any clear association with food intake. The patient denies any associated fever, chills, or anorexia.

PAST MEDICAL HISTORY:

1. _____ headaches.

2. Chronic lumbosacral back pain, status post repair of 2 herniated nucleus _____ at L4-5.

3. Cholelithiasis, status post cholecystectomy.

4. Four cesarean sections secondary to small pelvic outlet. These procedures were complicated by hemorrhage resulting in a total hysterectomy.

5. Multiple abdominal _____ noted on cholecystectomy.

PHYSICAL EXAMINATION: Vital signs: Pulse 81, _____ pressure 113/73, respirations 18, temperature 98.5, weight 242 pounds. General examination: The patient is alert and oriented × 3, in no apparent distress, morbidly obese. HEENT examination: Normocephalic and _____. Sclerae are _____. Neck: Supple. No thyromegaly. Cardiovascular examination: Regular rate and _____. No murmurs. Lungs: Clear to auscultation bilaterally. Back: Shows no spinal or CVA tenderness. Abdomen: Soft, obese, nondistended. There is mild tenderness to palpation in the epigastrium. No guarding, no masses. Normal _____ sounds are present throughout. Extremities: Show no cyanosis, _____, or edema.

(Continues)

PHYSICAL EXAMINATION *(Continued)*

DIAGNOSTIC STUDIES: Liver function studies showed a total bilirubin of 0.4 and alkaline _____ of 87, AST 16, ALT 36, and albumin of 3.8. _____ shows a white count of 6.8, hemoglobin 14, hematocrit 42.2, _____ 82.6, RDW 12.5, and platelets 149.

ASSESSMENT AND PLAN: Chronic right upper quadrant abdominal pain. Etiology unclear. The differential diagnosis includes pain from adhesions due to multiple abdominal surgeries, irritable bowel _____ versus type 3 sphincter of _____ dysfunction, or gastroparesis.

At this time, we will treat the patient symptomatically with Zelnorm 6 mg p.o. twice per day. We will perform a right upper _____ ultrasound to look for any evidence of biliary stones, and asked the patient to follow up in 5 to 6 weeks.

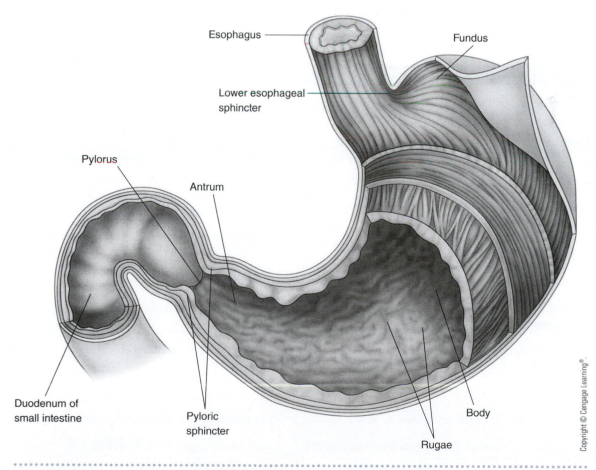

FIGURE 5-1 Structures of the Stomach

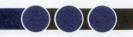

TASK 5-1B: MATCHING EXERCISE

Instructions: Match the following procedures in the column on the left with its definition from the column on the right.

1. _____ proctocolectomy	A. A procedure that involves bringing the end of the small intestine out through a stoma in the abdomen.
2. _____ cholecystectomy	B. A procedure in which the endoscope, along with x-ray imaging, is used to evaluate and treat problems in the bile ducts, gallbladder, and pancreas.
3. _____ colostomy	C. A procedure in which the endoscope is used to evaluate the stomach and duodenum.
4. _____ gastroduodenoscopy	D. The surgical removal of the entire colon and rectum.
5. _____ small bowel resection and anastomosis	E. A surgical procedure that generally includes the removal of the head of the pancreas, the duodenum, a portion of the stomach, and other nearby tissues.
6. _____ gastric emptying study	F. The surgical removal of the lower part of the stomach.
7. _____ Whipple procedure	G. The surgical removal of the gallbladder.
8. _____ Nissen fundoplication	H. A procedure to evaluate the rate at which food empties from the stomach and enters the small intestine.
9. _____ antrectomy	I. A surgical procedure in which the fundus of the stomach is wrapped around the lower part of the esophagus to prevent the backflow of acid into the esophagus.
10. _____ cholangiography	J. A procedure in which a diseased portion of bowel is removed and the two healthy ends are joined back together.

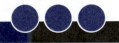

TASK 5-1C: MULTIPLE CHOICE EXERCISE

Instructions: Answer the following questions by circling the correct term in the choices (right) column.

Question	Choices
1. What is another name for upper GI series?	barium enema, barium swallow, laparoscopy
2. What is the middle part of the small intestine?	ileum, antrum, jejunum
3. What is the top portion of the colon extending from the hepatic flexure to the splenic flexure?	transverse colon, sigmoid colon, ascending colon
4. What is the vomiting of blood called?	hematemesis, melanoma, melena
5. What is the opening between the stomach and the small intestine?	antrum, pylorus, rectum
6. What is a bluish cast to the skin?	xanthoma, leukocytosis, cyanosis
7. What is the condition in which feces contain excessive fat?	steatohepatitis, steatorrhea, cirrhosis
8. What is another word for an enlarged liver?	pancreatitis, hepatomegaly, cardiomegaly
9. What is inflammation of the cells of the liver called?	pancreatitis, gastritis, hepatitis
10. What is another word for *hidden*?	occult, obtund, obese

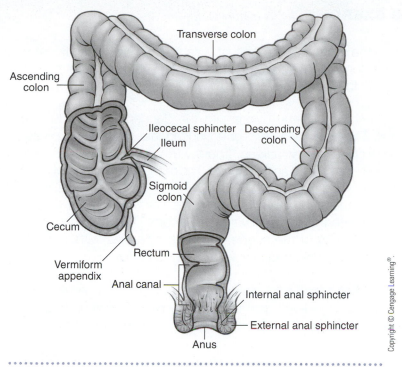

FIGURE 5-2 Structures of the Large Intestine

TASK 5-2: PROOFREADING EXERCISES

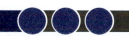

Instructions: The proofreading documents below are designed to challenge your proofreading and editing skills. The documents may contain missing demographic information, incorrect headings, misspelled words, misplaced punctuation, and other errors within the document. Read each report below and identify the error by circling the word. Then retype the document with the corrected text and formatting. When finished, proofread your work and save the document to your student disk using a different file name.

PROOFREADING EXERCISE 1

ENDOSCOPY NOTE

The patient underwent endoscopy because of a history of dysphasia with intractable esophageal symptoms. The risks complications, and alternatives were discussed with the patient.

MEDICATIONS:

1. Versed 5 mg.
2. Demerol 40 mg.

PROCEDURE: The olympus fiberoptic endoscope was inserted into the oropharynx and advanced into the esophagus without difficulty. The patient was seen to have a hiatus hernia. There was no obstruction there was no ring. Patient had mild esophagitis.

(Continues)

PROOFREADING EXERCISE 1 (Continued)

Biopsies were done. In the stomach, the patient was seen to have significant gastritis. Helibacter studies were done. The rest of the stomach was normal. A retrograde study was done to examine the fundus of the stomach, which was negative.

The scope was advanced through the pyloris into the duodenum. The duodenal bulb was seen to be normal. The scope was further advanced into the second portion of the duodenum, where the ampule was visualized. There was a small polyp arising from the mouth of the ampulla. This was snared and removed. The rest of the small bowl was normal.

The instrument was subsequently withdrawn from the duodenum into the stomach. The stomach was re-evaluated on withdrawal of the scope. The esophagus was then reevaluated on further withdraw of the scope. As the scope was withdrawn from the mouth, the vocal chords were evaluated and were seen to be lax.

SUMMARY: The patient has a hiatus hernia with esophagitis there is no evidence of an obstruction. The patient has significant gastritis. The duodenum was normal accept for a small polyp in the area of the ampulla, which was biopsied and removed.

We will plan to treat the patient aggressively with prilosec and Carafate therapy. The patient will call in a few days for the pathology report. All of this was discussed in detail with the patent and his family.

PROOFREADING EXERCISE 2

DISCHARGE SUMMARY

The patient is a 43-year-old male who has been known to us for over 20 years with Crohn's disease. He has had ileocolic resection many years ago for a perforation of his ilium secondary to blunt abdominal trauma.

Patient was doing relatively well until about 3 weeks prior to admission when he began to develop intermittent crampy abdominal pain. This was thought to be due to an exacerbation of his Crohn's disease. The patient was given prednisone and Asachol. He did not significantly improve. About one week prior to admission he began having chills, fever, and cramping pain. On the night of admission he developed acute abdominal pain, shaking chills, and a high fevers and was seen at the hospital.

PHYSICAL EXAMINATION: Remarkably benign. The abdomen was soft, bowl sounds were active. There were no masses, rebound, or guarding. The lungs were clear to ANP. The heart revealed normal sinus rhythm with a systolic ejection murmur. There was no lymph nodes. The neck was supple. The fundi were normal. The rectal exam revealed brown stool which was guaiac positive.

LABORATORY: The white count was 19000 with 75 percent neutrophils.

(Continues)

PROOFREADING EXERCISE 2 *(Continued)*

HOSPITAL COURSE: The patient was treated with intravenous steroids and intravenous antibiotics. The blood cultures the next day grew gram-negative organisms, which turned out to be Ecoli. The patient's white count remained elevated but gradually came down to normal, with a normal differential in the hospital. The patient was seen in consultation by an infectious disease consultant and was put on Flagyl and gentamicin because of his sepsis. His 6/60 was normal except for transient hyperkalemia secondary to the steroids and diuretic therapy given to him because of his edema. His 12/60 was normal except for an albumin of 2.5 and a calcium of 8.1. The magnesium level was normal. The amylase was normal. His gentamicin peak and troff levels were acceptable.

The patient was treated with several days of intraveneous antibiotics in the hospital and remained afebrile. A computed axial tomography scan of his abdomen suggested a possible abscess in the right midabdomen. This was followed up with several CT scans, which confirmed it. An upper G.I. series was done, which showed a collection in the right mid-abdomen just adjacent to his prior anastomosis, which communicated with the small bowel but appeared to be outside of the lumen. This was interpreted to be an abscess cavity which communicated with the gut and was filled with barium.

The patient will need surgical therapy. He is being discharged at this time in an improved condition on p.o. antibiotics. He will be readmitted to the hospital for surgery and resection of his inflammation bowel disease and the absess in a couple of days. If the patient develops any problems over the weekend, he will call us immediately. Surgery will be done by Dr. _____, who has operated on him in the past.

DISCHARGE MEDICATIONS:

1. Predisone 20 mg q.d.
2. Asacol 2 t.i.d.
3. Flagyl 500 mg t.i.d.
4. Cipro 5 mg po b.i.d.

We will follow the patient out of the hospital.

GASTROENTEROLOGY TRANSCRIPTION TIPS

1. When dictating, physicians may refer to the word *bilirubin* as "bili." You should avoid the use of this brief form and transcribe it in full, including its variations of *bilirubin*, *direct bilirubin*, and *total bilirubin*.

2. Sometimes doctors will refer to GI tests as "belly labs," which should not be transcribed as "bili labs." There is no such thing as a bili lab.

3. The plural of diverticulum is *diverticula*, NOT "diverticulae," "diverticulas," or "diverticuli," no matter how it is dictated.

4. A common surgical procedure option in gastroenterology is a *transjugular intrahepatic portosystemic shunt* (TIPS) procedure, which is performed to treat bleeding from varices in the esophagus or stomach as well as ascites in the abdomen caused by portal hypertension. Dictators may refer to this as a TIPS procedure, which sounds like "tips."

5. Do not confuse the homonyms *ilium* and *ileum*. The *ilium* refers to the bone located in the hip. The *ileum* is the part of the small intestine of the digestive system, between the duodenum and the colon, that absorbs digested food. Make sure you choose the correct term depending on the body structure or specialty that is the subject of the dictation. A helpful way to distinguish *ilium* from *ileum* is to think of the *e* in *ileum* being similar to the loops of the small and large intestines.

TASK 5-3:   CLOZE EXERCISES

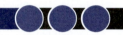

Instructions: The audio files for the following cloze exercises are located on the Premium website that accompanies this text (ISBN-13: 978-1-285-73537-5) at http://www.CengageBrain.com. If this is the first time you are registering your account, see the Preface for further instructions.

Once you are logged in to your account, locate the dictation file and Word document for the following cloze exercises. Open the audio file to be reviewed according to the exercise number indicated, along with its corresponding Word document. Listen to the dictation and read along with the text, filling in the missing words in the report by thinking critically and analytically about the context of the text you are reading. When finished, proofread your work and save the document according to your instructor's directions.

CLOZE EXERCISE 1: Operative Note_Report 5
Patient Name: Hsin Wu
Medical Record Number: 40907

CLOZE EXERCISE 2: Letter_Report 5118[2]
Patient Name: Lionel Rogers
Medical Record Number: 33505

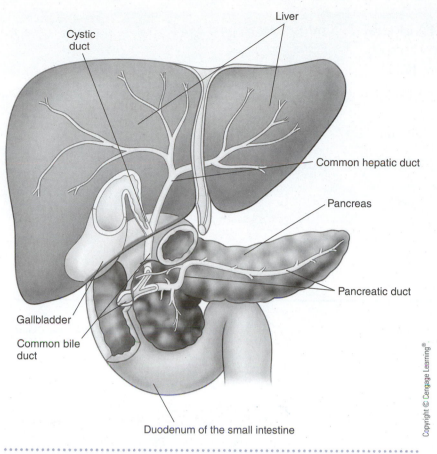

Cystic duct

Liver

Common hepatic duct

Pancreas

Pancreatic duct

Gallbladder

Common bile duct

Duodenum of the small intestine

Copyright © Cengage Learning®

FIGURE 5-3 Accessory Organs of the Digestive System

TASK 5-4: TRANSCRIPTION EXERCISES

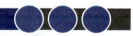

Instructions: The audio files for the following transcription exercises are located on the Premium website that accompanies this text (ISBN-13: 978-1-285-73537-5) at http://www.CengageBrain.com. If this is the first time you are registering your account, see the Preface for further instructions.

Once you are logged in to your account, locate and open the audio file to be transcribed according to the exercise number indicated and transcribe each report. Do not insert a heading into the document if the text requires a second page, but let the text wrap naturally to the second page and continue typing. Transcribe the reports using the formatting specifics indicated in the Document Formatting Guidelines located at the beginning of this book. When finished, proofread your work and save the document according to your instructor's directions.

TRANSCRIPTION EXERCISE 1: Progress Note_Report 5173[1]
Patient Name: Stuart Smith
Medical Record Number: 55711

TRANSCRIPTION EXERCISE 2: Operative Note_Report 4
Patient Name: Blake Brooks
Medical Record Number: 88091

TRANSCRIPTION EXERCISE 3: Endoscopy_Report 5132

Patient Name: Grant Parkinson

Medical Record Number: 17243

TRANSCRIPTION EXERCISE 4: Consultation, with Flexible Sigmoidoscopy_Report 5128

Patient Name: Betty Payne

Medical Record Number: 31790

TRANSCRIPTION EXERCISE 5: History and Physical, with EGD_Report 5161

Patient Name: Luke Jensen

Medical Record Number: 34562

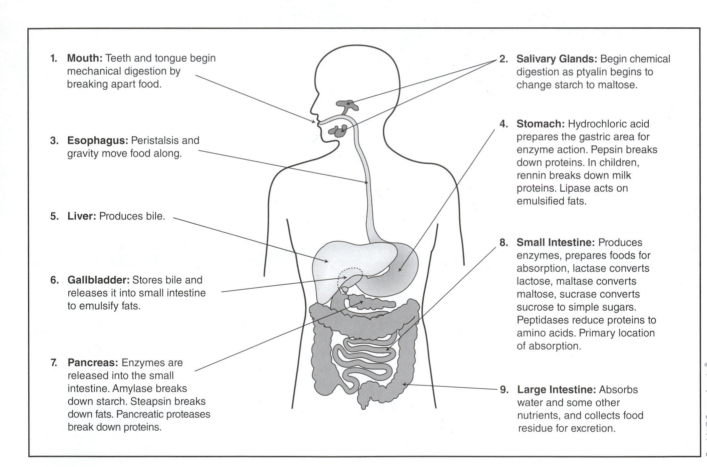

1. **Mouth:** Teeth and tongue begin mechanical digestion by breaking apart food.

2. **Salivary Glands:** Begin chemical digestion as ptyalin begins to change starch to maltose.

3. **Esophagus:** Peristalsis and gravity move food along.

4. **Stomach:** Hydrochloric acid prepares the gastric area for enzyme action. Pepsin breaks down proteins. In children, rennin breaks down milk proteins. Lipase acts on emulsified fats.

5. **Liver:** Produces bile.

6. **Gallbladder:** Stores bile and releases it into small intestine to emulsify fats.

7. **Pancreas:** Enzymes are released into the small intestine. Amylase breaks down starch. Steapsin breaks down fats. Pancreatic proteases break down proteins.

8. **Small Intestine:** Produces enzymes, prepares foods for absorption, lactase converts lactose, maltase converts maltose, sucrase converts sucrose to simple sugars. Peptidases reduce proteins to amino acids. Primary location of absorption.

9. **Large Intestine:** Absorbs water and some other nutrients, and collects food residue for excretion.

FIGURE 5-4 Overview of Digestion

TASK 5-5: SPEECH RECOGNITION EXERCISES
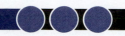

Instructions: The audio files for the following speech recognition exercises are located on the Premium website that accompanies this text (ISBN-13: 978-1-285-73537-5) at http://www.CengageBrain.com. If this is the first time you are registering your account, see the Preface for further instructions.

Once you are logged in to your account, locate the dictation file and Word document for the following speech recognition exercises. Open the audio file to be reviewed according to the exercise number indicated, along with its corresponding Word document. Listen to the dictation and read along with the text, making corrections to the text with regard to formatting, terminology, grammar, spelling, and punctuation. When finished, proofread your work and save the document according to your instructor's directions.

SRT EXERCISE 1: Operative Note_Report 2
Patient Name: Dorothy Daniels
Medical Record Number: 52539

SRT EXERCISE 2: Discharge Summary_Report 5145
Patient Name: Lisa Shaw
Medical Record Number: 97608

SRT EXERCISE 3: Letter_Report 5126[2]
Patient Name: Lincoln McFadden
Medical Record Number: 111820

SRT EXERCISE 4: Clinic Note_Report 4
Patient Name: Aman Shah
Medical Record Number: 688291

COMPUTER SOFTWARE TIPS

1. You can add misspelled words to Auto Correct instantly by right-clicking on the word that is flagged as misspelled. The **Edit** shortcut menu will appear. If Word has suggested an alternative, **AutoCorrect** will appear on the menu. Choose **AutoCorrect** and then select the correct version of the word from the submenu to create an Auto-Correct entry on the fly.

2. To see two parts of a document at the same time, from the **View** ribbon, choose **Split**. Click to place the split bar where you want to divide the document window. Now you can see both parts of the document, including separate vertical scroll bars, to navigate each part of the document. To restore the panes to a single window, from the **View** ribbon, choose **Remove Split**.

3. You can quickly activate the header or footer area in the document by double-clicking over the header or footer at the top or bottom of the document. Double-click in the document page area to turn off the header and footer areas.

4. To hide the white space between pages of a document, move the mouse to the area between pages of a document and double-click. To restore the white space, double-click on the dividing line between the pages.

5. To see paragraph marks and other hidden formatting symbols in a document, from the **Home** ribbon, use the **Show/Hide** button, which looks like a backward letter P.

GENERAL BOOK OF STYLE **TIPS**

1. Spell out nonmetric units of measure (ounce, pound, inch, foot, yard, mile, etc.). Do not use an apostrophe or quotation marks to indicate feet or inches in text. Do not put a comma or other punctuation between units of the same dimension.

    4 pounds

    5 ounces

    5 feet 4 inches (*not* 5'4" or 5 feet, 4 inches)

    Use a hyphen to join a number and a nonmetric unit of measure when they are used as an adjective preceding a noun.

    a 5-inch wound

    8-pound 5-ounce baby girl

2. The *Gram stain* is named after Hans Christian Gram, the Danish bacteriologist who originally devised it as a staining method used in the identification of bacteria. When transcribing Gram stain results, capitalize the word Gram.

    We ordered a Gram stain.

    Gram stain revealed a new species of bacteria. (*not* Gram's)

    However, when describing the Gram stain, the word is in lowercase with a hyphen.

    The specimen was gram-negative.

    The culture grew out gram-positive rods.

3. *Specific gravity* is a laboratory item often dictated in urinalysis findings. This value is expressed with four digits, with a decimal point placed between the first and second digits. Do not drop the final zero.

    Dictated: specific gravity ten twenty

    Transcribed: specific gravity 1.020

4. Do not start out a sentence with a number if at all possible. Spell out numbers that begin a sentence, or recast the sentence.

    Dictated: Fifteen days ago the patient was admitted to the outside facility.

    Transcribed: Fifteen days ago the patient was admitted to the outside facility.

    or

    Transcribed: The patient was admitted to the outside facility 15 days ago. (preferred)

5. Use hyphens when numbers are used with words as compound modifiers preceding nouns with English units of measure. Do not hyphenate compound modifiers if the unit of measure is an abbreviated metric unit.

    3-week history

    2-year-old female

    2-inch laceration

    but

    3 cm incision

    5 mg dosage

    5 × 3 × 2 cm mass

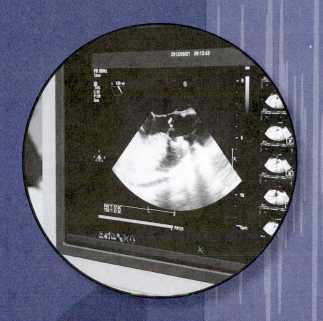

PROJECT 6

Obstetrics and Gynecology

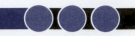

TASK 6-1A: TRUE/FALSE EXERCISE

Instructions: Read each statement and indicate whether it is true or false. If false, rewrite the sentence to make the statement true, replacing either the italicized term or the description/definition of the term contained in the sentence.

1. Statement: *Dysmenorrhea* is the complete absence of monthly menstrual periods.

   Answer: _____

   Correction, if false: _____

   _____

2. *Mastitis* is a postpartum inflammation of the breast.

   Answer: _____

   Correction, if false: _____

   _____

3. The presence of the *BRCA-1* gene does not increase a woman's risk of developing breast cancer.

   Answer: _____

   Correction, if false: _____

   _____

4. A *pediatrician* is a physician who specializes in the caring and treatment of newborns up to 28 days.

   Answer: _____

   Correction, if false: _____

   _____

5. A *pessary* is an appliance introduced into the vagina to support the uterus.

   Answer: _____

   Correction, if false: _____

   _____

6. *Cryosurgery* is the name of a procedure whereby liquid nitrogen is used to freeze a section of the cervix in order to destroy abnormal or precancerous cervical cells.

   Answer: _____

   Correction, if false: _____

   _____

7. The term *congenital* means "across or through the abdomen."

   Answer: _____

   Correction, if false: _____

   _____

8. The birth of an infant who dies before delivery is called a *neonate*.

   Answer: _____

   Correction, if false: _____

   _____

9. *Nulligravida* describes a woman's first menstrual period.

   Answer: _____

   Correction, if false: _____

   _____

10. The term *in vitro* means an artificial environment.

Answer: _____

Correction, if false: _____

_____

11. A procedure whereby both the ovaries and salpinges are removed is called *bilateral salpingo-oophorectomies*.

Answer: _____

Correction, if false: _____

_____

12. Irregular bleeding between menstrual periods is referred to as *menorrhagia*.

Answer: _____

Correction, if false: _____

_____

13. A *quad marker screen* is a blood test to determine the risk of having a baby with a birth defect.

Answer: _____

Correction, if false: _____

_____

14. A *LEEP* procedure is used to remove endocervical tissue using a curette.

Answer: _____

Correction, if false: _____

_____

15. A woman may undergo a *vulvectomy* to prevent her from having any more children.

Answer: _____

Correction, if false: _____

_____

TASK 6-1B: MEDICAL WORD BUILDING EXERCISE

Instructions: Using the given list of suffixes, build a medical term for the meaning given.

| -plasty | -graphy | -rrhea | -osis | -metry |
| -pexy | -ectomy | -scopy | -itis | -dynia |

1. Surgical repair of the breast.   _____

2. Incision into the amniotic sac.   _____

3. Visual inspection of the tissues of the cervix and vagina.   _____

4. Surgical excision of the uterus.   _____

5. Surgical removal of myomas.   _____

6. Inflammation of the salpinx.   _____

7. Pain in the breast. _____

8. Difficult or painful menstruation _____

9. Inflammation of the endometrium _____

10. Surgical fixation of the vagina _____

TASK 6-1C: MATCHING EXERCISE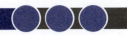

Instructions: Match the medical condition in the left column with its definition in the right column.

1. _____ cervical dysplasia

2. _____ menopause

3. _____ amenorrhea

4. _____ dystocia

5. _____ vulvodynia

6. _____ dyspareunia

7. _____ menometrorrhagia

8. _____ fibromyoma

9. _____ preeclampsia

10. _____ endometriosis

11. _____ atresia

12. _____ salpingitis

13. _____ microcephaly

14. _____ uterine prolapse

15. _____ omphalocele

A. Chronic vulvar discomfort.

B. Development of hypertension with proteinuria, edema, or both, due to pregnancy.

C. Congenital absence of a normal opening, such as the esophagus or anus.

D. Protrusion of the uterus into or through the vagina.

E. Congenital herniation at the umbilical cord.

F. The development of abnormal cells in the lining of the cervix.

G. Pain during sexual intercourse.

H. The permanent cessation of menses.

I. A congenital condition characterized by an abnormally small head.

J. The presence of endometrial tissue somewhere other than in the lining of the uterus.

K. Irregular and excessive menstrual bleeding.

L. A benign growth that develops from the smooth muscular tissue of the uterus.

M. Inflammation of the salpinx.

N. The absence of menstrual bleeding.

O. Difficult childbirth.

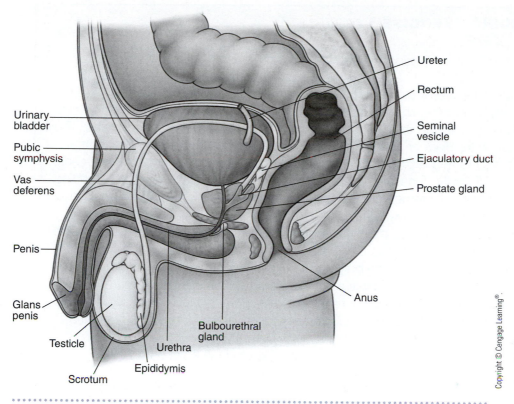

FIGURE 6-1 The Male Reproductive System

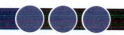

TASK 6-2: PROOFREADING EXERCISES

Instructions: The proofreading documents below are designed to challenge your proofreading and editing skills. The documents may contain missing demographic information, incorrect headings, misspelled words, misplaced punctuation, and other errors within the document. Read each report below and identify the error by circling the word. Then retype the document with the corrected text and formatting. When finished, proofread your work and save the document to your student disk using a different file name.

PROOFREADING EXERCISE 1

SUBJECTIVE: The patient is a 35-year-old nuligravida, status post first attempt at invitro fertilization and embryo transfer, who comes in for salene infusion sonography and to discuss further management plans. Full written informed consent was obtained to proceed with saline infusion sonography with this patient today.

OBJECTIVE: The patient is an alert and oriented caucasian female in no acute distress. Skin Without rashes or lesions. Neck: Without thyromegaly. Nodes were negative. Lungs were clear to auscultation and percussion. Heart: Regular sinus rhythm. No murmurs. Breast: Without masses, galactorea, or retraction. Axillary nodes were negative. Abdomen: No hepatosplenomegaly. No CVA tenderness. No masses. Inguinal nodes were negative. Pelvic exam revealed normal external genitalia without lesions and normal vagina without lesions. Cervix was posterior. No lesions was noted. Nontender. Uterus was deeply antiverted, almost anteflexed, small size, mobile. Adnexa without masses or tenderness. Cul de sac was without nodularity.

(Continues)

PROOFREADING EXERCISE 1 *(Continued)*

At this point, saline infusion sonography was performed. First, a sterile speculum was placed in the vagina. Next, the cervix was cleansed with Betadine. Tenaculum was placed in the anterior lip of the cervix and a trail transfer was performed with abdominal ultrasound scan revealing a deeply anteverted, almost anteflexed uterus with impaction. The wallace catheter was passed through the endocervical canal to a depth of 7-1/2 centimetrs. The patient will require a full bladder at the time of the actual embryo transfer. At this point, the catheter was removed and a Cook catheter was passed through the endocervical canal into the endometrial cavity. Tenaculum was removed from the vagina. No gross bleeding was noted. Speculum was removed from the vagina and vaginal probe was inserted in the vagina after first placing a condom over the vagina probe. Saline infusion sonography was performed by attaching a 60-mL sterile normal saline containing syringe. The uterine fundus appears somewhat distorted by about a one- cm endometrial polyp, very thick endometrium measuring 8.7 mm. The polyp was noticeable both in the saggital as well as transverse views of the endometrium. In the anterior portion of the uterus intramurally. There was evidence of a small fibroid or focus of adenomyosis, both ovaries were visualized and appeared grossly normal with multiple follicular cysts noted. No evidence of endometriosis was seen. Saline infusion sonography was ended. The catheter was removed from the vagina. The vaginal probe was removed. The patient tolerated the procedure well.

ASSESSMENT: Endometrial polyps visualized today under saline infusion sonography. The patient has a history of primary infertile.

I reviewed with this patient the present findings as well as treatment options. We discussed doing nothing, medical suppressed, surgical evaluation and treatment vs. proceeding with in vitro fertilization and embryo transfer attempt number 2. The patient will discuss with her husband and will then make another appointment for further consultation.

PLAN: The patient is to make a decision based on her discussion of the present findings with her husband. She will then consult with us at a separte time.

PROOFREADING EXERCISE 2

SUBJECTIVE: The patient is a 26-year-old, G2, P0, 0-2-0, who has been followed by the Gyn Clinic because of a possible etopic pregnancy. She had a beta HCG drawn on October 12, 2006, which was 77. At that time, she had transvaginal ultrasound done, which showed a 3.5×2.6 cm, left adnexal mass with positive free fluid. She had a followup ultrasound done and the left adnexa was 2.88×2.55 cm with no fluid in the pelvis. She had a Beta HCG drawn today, which was 28. The patient denies any fever, chills, nausea, vomiting, abdominal pain, or vaginal bleeding. She denies any other symptoms.

PHYSICAL EXAMINATION: Vital signs The patient is 5 foot, 9 inches tall, 129 pounds, her blood pressure is 110/80.

GENERAL: No acute distress.

CARDIOVASCULAR: Regular rate and rhythm.

(Continues)

PROOFREADING EXERCISE 2 *(Continued)*

LUNGS: Clear to auscultation bilaterally.

ABDOMINAL: Soft, nontender, nondistended. No rebound, no guarding.

EXTREMITIES: Without clubbing, cyanosis, or edema.

ASSESSMENT AND PLAN: The patient is a 26-year-old, G2, P0-0-2-0, with possible ectopic versus missed ab. The patient was instructed to followup in 1 week for a repeat beta HCG. We will call her with the results. She was also instructed to follow up sooner if she had any abdominal pain, nausea, vomiting, fever, chills, or vaginal bleding. She states that she understands.

 # OBSTETRICS AND GYNECOLOGY TRANSCRIPTION **TIPS**

1. During a gynecologic examination, a physician may say, "BUS (pronounced like "bus") is negative," referring to the abbreviation for the *Bartholin, urethra,* and *Skene glands* located in that area of the vulva. Another phrase used in dictation sounds like "egg-bus is negative." The abbreviation used is EG/BUS, which stands for *external genitalia/ Bartholin, urethral, and Skene* (glands).

2. *Adnexa* are appendages or adjunct parts. This word is used in the plural, even when physicians are only referring to one side; thus, do not transcribe this word in the singular.

3. Be careful when typing the term *fetal*, relating to a fetus, that you do not accidentally type *fecal*,

relating to feces. A spell checker would not pick up this glaring error.

4. Dictators often mispronounce the word *cornua*, which is the horn of the uterus where the fallopian tubes join the uterine cavity, as sounding like *cornea*, which is the transparent outer part of the eye.

5. Pediatricians are present during the birth of a baby to examine and care for the baby immediately after it is born. Dictators will often refer to these physicians as "peds" (pronounced like "peeds") and say, for example, "the infant was handed off to waiting peds." Use the word *pediatricians* when transcribing this slang expression.

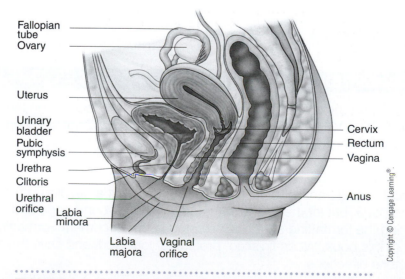

FIGURE 6-2 The Female Reproductive System

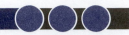

TASK 6-3: CLOZE EXERCISES

Instructions: The audio files for the following cloze exercises are located on the Premium website that accompanies this text (ISBN-13: 978-1-285-73537-5) at http://www.CengageBrain.com. If this is the first time you are registering your account, see the Preface for further instructions.

Once you are logged in to your account, locate the dictation file and Word document for the following cloze exercises. Open the audio file to be reviewed according to the exercise number indicated, along with its corresponding Word document. Listen to the dictation and read along with the text, filling in the missing words in the report by thinking critically and analytically about the context of the text you are reading. When finished, proofread your work and save the document according to your instructor's directions.

CLOZE EXERCISE 1: Bilateral Mammograms_Report 3267
Patient Name: Rosa Nunez
Medical Record Number: 87691

CLOZE EXERCISE 2: Clinic Note_Report 6
Patient Name: Wanda Lowe
Medical Record Number: 44736

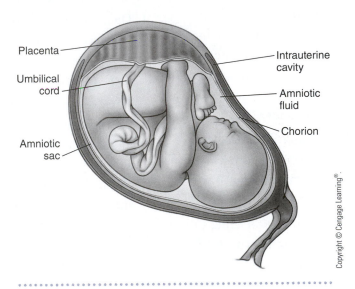

FIGURE 6-3 A Normal Pregnant Uterus

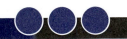

TASK 6-4: TRANSCRIPTION EXERCISES

Instructions: The audio files for the following transcription exercises are located on the Premium website that accompanies this text (ISBN-13: 978-1-285-73537-5) at http://www.CengageBrain.com. If this is the first time you are registering your account, see the Preface for further instructions.

Once you are logged in to your account, locate and open the audio file to be transcribed according to the exercise number indicated and transcribe each report. Do not insert a heading into the document if the text requires a second page, but let the text wrap naturally to the second page and continue typing. Transcribe the reports using the formatting specifics indicated in the Document Formatting Guidelines located at the beginning of this book. When finished, proofread your work and save the document according to your instructor's directions.

TRANSCRIPTION EXERCISE 1: **Clinic Note_Report 8**
Patient Name: Louise Craig
Medical Record Number: 48309

TRANSCRIPTION EXERCISE 2: **Operative Note_Report 3**
Patient Name: Nicole Bowman
Medical Record Number: 11298

TRANSCRIPTION EXERCISE 3: **Discharge Summary_Report 3**
Patient Name: Chen Kim
Medical Record Number: 23331

TRANSCRIPTION EXERCISE 4: **Operative Note_Report 13**
Patient Name: Paula Gregory
Medical Record Number: 59941

TRANSCRIPTION EXERCISE 5: **Discharge Summary_Report 4**
Patient Name: Jayson Cole
Medical Record Number: 75402

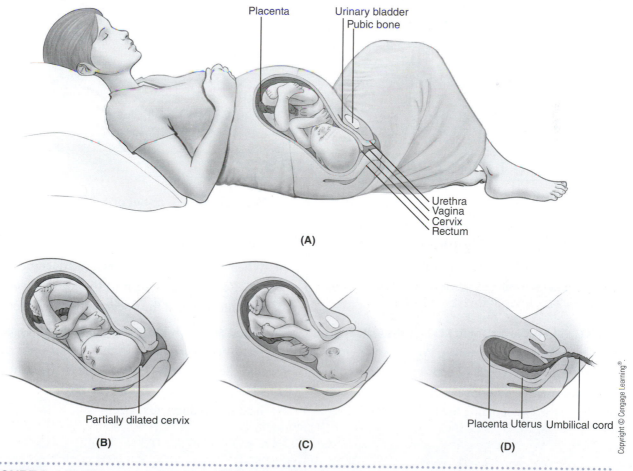

FIGURE 6-4 The Stages of Labor. (A) Position of the Fetus Before Labor. (B) First Stage of Labor, Cervical Dilation. (C) Second Stage of Labor, Fetal Delivery. (D) Third Stage of Labor, Delivery of the Placenta and Fetal Membranes.

TASK 6-5: SPEECH RECOGNITION EXERCISES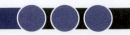

Instructions: The audio files for the following speech recognition exercises are located on the Premium website that accompanies this text (ISBN-13: 978-1-285-73537-5) at http://www.CengageBrain.com. If this is the first time you are registering your account, see the Preface for further instructions.

Once you are logged in to your account, locate the dictation file and Word document for the following speech recognition exercises. Open the audio file to be reviewed according to the exercise number indicated, along with its corresponding Word document. Listen to the dictation and read along with the text, making corrections to the text with regard to formatting, terminology, grammar, spelling, and punctuation. When finished, proofread your work and save the document according to your instructor's directions.

SRT EXERCISE 1: Left Breast Sonogram_Report 3223
Patient Name: Kelly Fowler
Medical Record Number: 55311

SRT EXERCISE 2: Clinic Note_Report 4
Patient Name: Connie Parks
Medical Record Number: 16586

SRT EXERCISE 3: Clinic Note_Report 37
Patient Name: Rashonda Dillingham
Medical Record Number: 77290

SRT EXERCISE 4: Clinic Note_Report 63
Patient Name: Sharla Raines
Medical Record Number: 211001

 COMPUTER SOFTWARE **TIPS**

1. You can quickly insert an em dash or en dash into a document using keyboard shortcuts. Type **CTRL + ALT + −** (the minus key on the numeric keypad) for the em dash or **CTRL + −** (the minus sign on the numeric keypad) for the en dash.

2. **CTRL + O** is the common keyboard shortcut for the Open command. However, Word also retained the previous **CTRL + F12** shortcut leftover from early versions of Windows. Thus both shortcuts will open the Open dialog box.

3. You can zoom in or out of a document by holding down the **CTRL** key while rotating the mouse wheel back and forth.

4. When you open a previously saved document, press **SHIFT + F5** to return to the location you were working on when the document was last closed.

5. If you simply want to increase the font size of a word or selected text, highlight the word or text and click the **Grow Font** button to the right of the Font Size drop-down list. The Shrink Font button next to it reduces text size.

OBSTETRICS AND GYNECOLOGY BOOK OF STYLE TIPS

1. There are three separate stages of labor, which are expressed with the word *stage* in lowercase letters and arabic numerals.

   The patient was admitted to the hospital in stage 2 labor.

2. The cervix goes through the process of *dilation* and *effacement* during labor. *Dilation* is measured and expressed in centimeters (0 cm to 10 cm). *Effacement*, or thinning, of the cervix is the process by which the cervix prepares for delivery, and is expressed as a percentage, from 0% to 100%.

   The patient was examined and her cervix was found to be 2 cm dilated and 50% effaced.

3. When transcribing *Apgar scores*, type ratings with arabic numerals and write out numbers related to minutes.

   Apgar scores were 8 at one minute and 9 at five minutes.

4. The *Tanner system* is used to classify sexual maturity during puberty in both males and females. The classification is expressed with Tanner in initial caps followed by lowercase "stage" and arabic numerals.

   Examination of the patient showed she was a Tanner stage 2.

5. CIN is an acronym for *cervical intraepithelial neoplasia* and is used to describe the level of precancerous cells in the cervix. This value is expressed with arabic numerals from grade 1 (least severe) to grade 3 (most severe) with a hyphen placed between CIN and the numeral.

   CIN-1, CIN-2, CIN-3

   or

   CIN grade 1, CIN grade 2, CIN grade 3

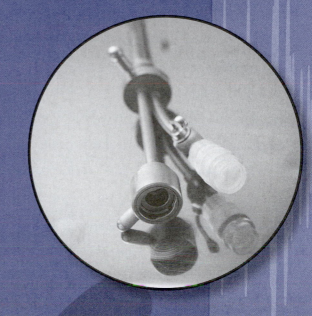

PROJECT 7

Urology

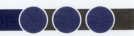

TASK 7-1A: SOUNDALIKE TERM REVIEW EXERCISE

Instructions: Circle the correct urologic term in the following sentences.

1. The patient underwent a (**urodynamic/urethroscopic**) study to evaluate how her body stores and releases urine.

2. Another name for a kidney stone is (**calculus, calcium**).

3. (**Creatine, creatinine**) is a component of urine.

4. The (**urethra, ureter**) connects the kidney to the urinary bladder.

5. The patient complained of (**anuria, dysuria**), or difficulty urinating.

6. The decreased capacity of the bladder due to aging can result in (**nocardia, nocturia**).

7. The adjective form for the word *bladder* is (**vesical, vesicle**).

8. Polycystic kidney disease can cause cysts that interfere with (**necrotic/nephron**) function.

9. A (**cystocele/cystogram**) causes the bladder to droop into the vagina.

10. The duct at the tip of each renal pyramid is called a (**callus, calix**).

11. The kidneys remove (**urea, urine**) from the blood.

12. The patient has undergone chemotherapy (**installation, instillation**) procedures within the bladder to treat his transitional cell carcinoma.

13. A Foley (**catheter, cautery**) was placed into the patient's bladder to assist with urination.

14. She has (**neurologic, neurogenic**) bladder, which requires her to self-catheterize.

15. He was diagnosed with a type of kidney stone known as a stag horn (**calculate, calculus**).

TASK 7-1B: FILL IN THE BLANKS EXERCISE

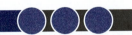

Instructions: Read the following clinic note and fill in the blanks in the record with the terms listed, relying on the context provided by the sentence to make your choices. Each term should be used only once.

red blood cells	particulate	sigmoidoscopy
fistulae	pneumaturia	carcinoma
etiology	pyelogram	barium
cystourethrogram	prostate	diverticulitis
urgency	colon	sphincter

HISTORY AND PHYSICAL EXAMINATION

HISTORY OF PRESENT ILLNESS: A 71-year-old male presents to the office with a chief complaint of passing air through his urine _____. He also states that he is passing _____ material in the urine as well. He has slight frequency and _____, good urinary control, and nocturia 1 to 2 times.

(Continues)

HISTORY AND PHYSICAL EXAMINATION *(Continued)*

PAST MEDICAL HISTORY: He has diverticulosis, with several episodes of
_____ over the last several years. Otherwise, his health is reasonably good.

MEDICATION: He basically takes no medication.

PHYSICAL EXAMINATION: Abdomen: Negative abdomen, with no tenderness or masses. Genitalia: Normal, with normal scrotal contents, normal penis, and no hernias. Rectal: His _____ is smooth, flat, nontender, without nodules. Normal _____ tone.

LABORATORY DATA: Urinalysis is loaded with pus, bacteria, and _____. Cultures pending.

IMPRESSION: Pneumaturia is the result of gas-forming bacteria or colovesical _____, usually from diverticulitis, or colon _____.

PLAN: Voiding _____ and cystourethroscopy to determine _____ of the pneumaturia. Will also do an upper tract evaluation with an intravenous _____.

In addition, we will refer to a general surgeon to do a _____/colonoscopy and _____ enema. More likely than not he has a colovesical fistula secondary to diverticular disease or carcinoma of the _____.

TASK 7-1C: MULTIPLE CHOICE EXERCISE

Instructions: Circle the correct medical term for the definition given.

1. A surgical procedure to secure the kidney in place.
   nephrolysis   nephrotripsy   nephropexy

2. Involuntary urination.
   enuresis   dysuria   nocturia

3. A stone in the ureter.
   urethrocele   ureterolithiasis   ureterosepsis

4. The process of removing impurities from the blood when the kidneys are unable to do so.
   diuresis   hemodialysis   nephroplasty

5. The absence of urine.
   anuria   dysuria   polyuria

6. A radiographic image of the bladder.
   nephrogram   cystogram   renogram

7. Destruction of living tissue with an electric spark, commonly used in bladder surgery.

   fulguration　　　　　cryoablation　　　　　ureterolysis

8. Creation of an artificial opening in the kidney.

   renostomy　　　　　meatotomy　　　　　nephrostomy

9. Sudden stoppage of urine formation.

   urinary suppression　　　incontinence　　　　enuresis

10. A tumor of the kidney.

    pyeloma　　　　　nephroma　　　　　cystoma

11. Protrusion of a ureter.

    ureterostenosis　　　ureteritis　　　　　ureterocele

12. A stone in the bladder.

    cystitis　　　　　cystolith　　　　　cystocele

13. Difficult or painful urination.

    dysuria　　　　　nocturia　　　　　anuria

14. A physician who studies and treats conditions of the urinary tract.

    nephrologist　　　　urologist　　　　　gastroenterologist

15. Excessive urea and nitrogenous substances in the blood.

    nocturia　　　　　azotemia　　　　　pyuria

TASK 7-2: PROOFREADING EXERCISES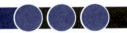

Instructions: The proofreading documents below are designed to challenge your proofreading and editing skills. The documents may contain missing demographic information, incorrect headings, misspelled words, misplaced punctuation, and other errors within the document. Read each report below and identify the error by circling the word. Then retype the document with the corrected text and formatting. When finished, proofread your work and save the document to your student disk using a different file name.

PROOFREADING EXERCISE 1

OPERATIVE REPORT

OPERATION PERFORMED: Bilateral vastectomy.

OPERATIVE TECHNIQUE: Patient was prepped and draped in the usual supine position using betadine. The vas on both sides were palpitated and brought towards the midline anterior scrotum. Using special vas clamps, the vas on the left side was grasped under the skin, a 1-inch vertical incision was made over the vaz, and the vas was then grasped with Alice clamps. Approximately 2 mL of anesthesia was injected under the skin prior to the incision, and an additional 2 cc of 1% Xylocaine was injected into the proximal and distal vas as well. With adequate anesthesia, the tissue over the vas on the left side was incised until the vas was easily seen. The vas deferens on the right was then grasped with towel clip, and the surrounding tissue was dissected off the vas itself. The vas deferens was then clamped proximally and distally, and the intervening 1.5 inches was incised and removed. Using a hyfrecator, the proximal and distal vas lumens were cauterized, and bleeding points, as well, were cauterized. Having completed the left-sided vasectomy, the vas was allowed to fall back into the scrotal compartment,

(Continues)

PROOFREADING EXERCISE 1 *(Continued)*

and through the same incision the right vas was grasped with clamps and infiltrated with several mL's of 1% Xylocaine.

The tissue over the vas was incised using knife technique, and the tissue was then disected off a 1-1/2-inch segment of the vas deferens. The proximal and distal vas was clamped, and the intervening 1-1/2-inch segment was incized and removed. Using the hyfrecator the proximal and distal lumens of the vas were cauterized as well as several bleeding points. On this particular side, a three-0 plain suture was utilized to cover over the proximal vas since the vas did not retract as on the left side. Having done the above, the scrotum was pulled down and the vas retracted into the right scrotal compartment.

No bleeding was noted, and the skin was then closed with a horizontal mattress suture of 3-0 plane. The scrotum was then cleaned with peroxide, and a fluf-type dressing with an athletic supporter was then utilized to cover the wound and give support to the scrotum. The patient was then cleaned up and discharged from the office with Tylenol #4, #10 every 3 to 6 hours prn pain.

She will return to the office in approximately 2 weeks for routine follow up. He is well aware that he is not sterile until his sperm count is 0. He will obtain his first sperm count in approximately one month.

PROOFREADING EXERCISE 2

PROCEDURE REPORT

A 17 year old female with recurrent urinary tract infections who was found on intravenous pyelogram to have dilatation of both urethras. Her recurrent infections have been a combination of Klebsiella urinary tract infections with E. koli urinary tract infections. A recurrent urinary tract infection work up was done today, including a voiding cystourethrogram and cystourethroscopy.

The voiding cystoureterogram shows bilateral ureterovesicle reflux, with contrast material visualized in both renal pelvises and significant dilatation of both ureters during the voiding phase. There is a mild to moderate post void residual due to contrast material trickling back into the bladder after the bladder has emptied.

Cystourethroscopy was performed. It showed a tight urethra, but more importantly a poorly formed vesical trigon, with golf hole ureteral orifices bilaterally and laterally placed. No doubt this young lady has a significant congenital anomaly of the ureterovesical junction, with bilateral reflux hydroureter and reflux of bladder material into the renal pelvis.

After discussion with the patient and explaining to her that she has a significant cogenital anomaly that will not respond to conservative treatments and will not disappear based upon her age, bilateral ureterovesical reimplantation would be the treatment of choice. We will schedule her for bilateral vesicle reimplantation in the near future, but in the meantime will maintain on urosuppressive agents, macrobid 100 mg po. b.id.

She is aware that she must maintain herself on urosuppresive agents until definitive surgicle repair can be completed.

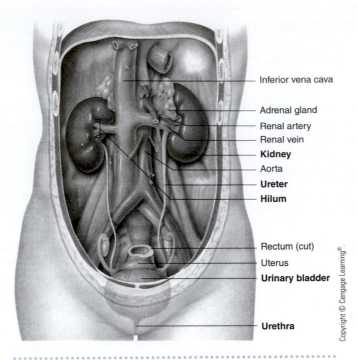

FIGURE 7-1 The Organs of the Urinary System of a Female

 # UROLOGY TRANSCRIPTION **TIPS**

1. Sometimes physicians will shorten the names of the drugs vancomycin, ampicillin, and gentamicin in dictation, respectively, as "vanc," "amp," and "gent." As with other shortened forms of words, spell out these terms when transcribing the names of these medications.

2. When patients with chronic renal failure develop more acute symptoms, physicians refer to this as *acute-on-chronic* renal failure. Do not transcribe this as "acute and chronic."

3. Kidney transplantation is the process of placing a healthy kidney from one person (the donor) into the body of another person (the recipient). The word "donor" is singular, not possessive, when transcribing either the location where the donated kidney is taken (the "donor site") or the donated kidney itself ("the donor kidney").

4. Do not mistake the term *ureter* with *urethra*. The *ureters*, one exiting from each kidney, are muscular tubes that pass urine from the kidneys to the bladder. The *urethra* is a tube that conveys urine from the bladder to the outside of the body. When you hear a dictator referring to the left or the right, the term is *ureter*, not *urethra*.

5. Do not mistranscribe the term *double-J ureteral stent* as "J and J ureteral stent." The ends of the double-J stent actually look like the letter J, hence the name *double-J stent*. Therefore, "J and J," "J&J," and "JJ" are all incorrect transcriptions of this stent.

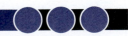

TASK 7-3: CLOZE EXERCISES

Instructions: The audio files for the following cloze exercises are located on the Premium website that accompanies this text (ISBN-13: 978-1-285-73537-5) at http://www.CengageBrain.com. If this is the first time you are registering your account, see the Preface for further instructions.

Once you are logged in to your account, locate the dictation file and Word document for the following cloze exercises. Open the audio file to be reviewed according to the exercise number indicated, along with its corresponding Word document. Listen to the dictation and read along with the text, filling in the missing words in the report by thinking critically and analytically about the context of the text you are reading. When finished, proofread your work and save the document according to your instructor's directions.

CLOZE EXERCISE 1: Progress Note_Report 2130
Patient Name: Marilyn Wade
Medical Record Number: 07469

CLOZE EXERCISE 2: Progress Note_Report 2183
Patient Name: John Wolff
Medical Record Number: 02183

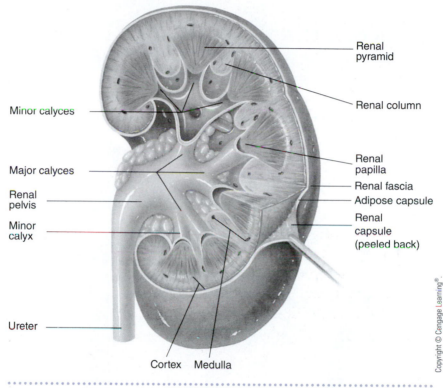

Renal
pyramid

Renal column

Minor calyces

Renal
papilla

Major calyces

Renal fascia
Adipose capsule

Renal
pelvis

Renal
capsule
(peeled back)

Minor
calyx

Ureter

Cortex Medulla

FIGURE 7-2 The Structure of the Kidney

TASK 7-4: TRANSCRIPTION EXERCISES

Instructions: The audio files for the following transcription exercises are located on the Premium website that accompanies this text (ISBN-13: 978-1-285-73537-5) at http://www.CengageBrain.com. If this is the first time you are registering your account, see the Preface for further instructions.

Once you are logged in to your account, locate and open the audio file to be transcribed according to the exercise number indicated and transcribe each report. Do not insert a heading into the document if the text requires a second page, but let the text wrap naturally to the second page and continue typing. Transcribe the reports using the formatting specifics indicated in the Document Formatting Guidelines located at the beginning of this book. When finished, proofread your work and save the document according to your instructor's directions.

TRANSCRIPTION EXERCISE 1: **History and Physical_Report 2133**
Patient Name: Vincent Jordan
Medical Record Number: 05354

TRANSCRIPTION EXERCISE 2: **Letter_Report 2174**
Patient Name: Graham Ross
Medical Record Number: 14871

TRANSCRIPTION EXERCISE 3: **Abdominal X-ray_Report 3143**
Patient Name: Julie Reed
Medical Record Number: 85319

TRANSCRIPTION EXERCISE 4: **Excretory Urogram_Report 3180**
Patient Name: Raphael Morales
Medical Record Number: 98265

TRANSCRIPTION EXERCISE 5: **Clinic Note_Report 11**
Patient Name: David Ellis
Medical Record Number: 13013

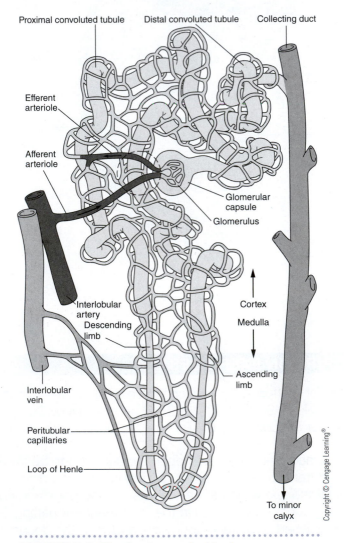

FIGURE 7-3 The Anatomy of a Nephron

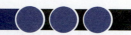

TASK 7-5:   SPEECH RECOGNITION EXERCISES

Instructions: The audio files for the following speech recognition exercises are located on the Premium website that accompanies this text (ISBN-13: 978-1-285-73537-5) at http://www.CengageBrain.com. If this is the first time you are registering your account, see the Preface for further instructions.

Once you are logged in to your account, locate the dictation file and Word document for the following speech recognition exercises. Open the audio file to be reviewed according to the exercise number indicated, along with its corresponding Word document. Listen to the dictation and read along with the text, making corrections to the text with regard to formatting, terminology, grammar, spelling, and punctuation. When finished, proofread your work and save the document according to your instructor's directions.

SRT EXERCISE 1: History and Physical_Report 2118
Patient Name: Gus Fisher
Medical Record Number: 44480

SRT EXERCISE 2: Letter_Report 2140
Patient Name: Tammy Hopkins
Medical Record Number: 95493

SRT EXERCISE 3: Progress Note_Report 2138
Patient Name: Sidney Ahlert
Medical Record Number: 038844

SRT EXERCISE 4: Progress Note_Report 2143
Patient Name: Grace Brazier
Medical Record Number: 229101

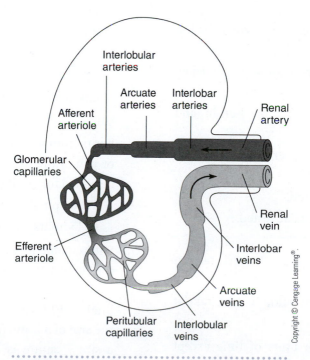

FIGURE 7-4 Blood Flow Through the Kidney

COMPUTER SOFTWARE **TIPS**

1. To find a meaning of a word quickly, simply highlight the word and right-click the mouse. A window opens to the right where you can see the meaning from the Encarta Dictionary. The **All Reference Books** drop-down box gives you other choices as well, including the thesaurus, translation, and other research websites.

2. Create a desktop shortcut to your document from your file list by right-clicking on the name of the document and choosing **Send To** and **Desktop (Create Shortcut)**. A shortcut for that document or file appears on your desktop.

3. To quickly remove character formatting, such as bold, italic, or underline, and reset the text back to the normal style, select the text and press **CTRL + SPACEBAR**. To reset paragraph formatting, such as tabs and indents, back to the normal style press **CTRL + Q**.

4. You can quickly change the case of text from Title to UPPERCASE to lowercase by selecting the text and pressing **SHIFT + F3**. Each time you press **SHIFT + F3**, the case will change.

5. Use line numbering to help you refer to specific parts of your document. Open the **Page Layout** ribbon. In the **Page Setup** section, click **Line Numbers** and select your options from the popup menu.

GENERAL BOOK OF STYLE **TIPS**

1. Avoid the use of contractions in the medical record, even if dictated, *except in direct quotations.* When possible, expand abbreviations that contain contractions, particularly when they represent slang or coined terms.

> Dictated: The patient can't recall when she last had a Pap smear.
>
> Transcribed: The patient cannot recall when she last had a Pap smear.
>
> Dictated: The patient OD'd on heroin and alcohol.
>
> Transcribed: The patient overdosed on heroin and alcohol.
>
> Dictated: Stool was guaiac'd.
>
> Transcribed: Stool was guaiac tested.
>
> *but*
>
> Dictated: The patient said, "I can't take it anymore."
>
> Transcribed: The patient said, "I can't take it anymore."

2. Do not abbreviate English units of time except when using a slash. Do not use periods with such abbreviations.

> The patient is 5 days old.
>
> He will return in 3 weeks for followup.
>
> The patient was given fentanyl 50 mcg/hour for severe pain.
>
> Do not add "00" for on-the-hour expressions.
>
> 8:15 a.m.
>
> 8 a.m. or 8 o'clock in the morning.
>
> *not*
>
> 8:00 a.m. or 8:00 o'clock

When transcribing military time, do not separate hours from minutes with a colon. Do not use a.m. or p.m. If the word "hours" is not dictated, it may be added for clarity.

> 1300 hours
>
> 0845 hours

3. Suture come in various sizes. The larger the size, the smaller the size of the suture. The sizes range from 00 (very large, about the size of large fishing line) to 10-0 (or "ten zeros" and very tiny, about the size of a human hair). Therefore, for example, a size 7 suture is larger than a size 7-0 suture. When transcribing suture sizes, use 0 or 1-0 for single-aught sutures. Use the "digit hyphen zero"

style to express sizes 2-0 through 11-0. Express sizes 1 through 7 with whole numbers. Place the # symbol before the size if the word "number" is dictated.

> 1-0 nylon or 0 nylon
>
> 2-0 nylon, *not* 00 nylon
>
> 4-0 Vicryl, *not* 0000 Vicryl
>
> Dictated: The skin was closed with number 2-0 Vicryl sutures.
>
> Transcribed: The skin was closed with #2-0 Vicryl sutures.

4. When transcribing fractions, express them with numerals when they are followed by a *nonmetric* value. Use decimals with metric values.

> The laceration measured 2-1/2 inches.
>
> She had chest pain approximately 1-1/2 hours prior to admission.
>
> *but*
>
> The wound measured 1.5 cm.
>
> *not*
>
> The wound measured 1-1/2 cm.

Spell out fractions when they are *not* followed by any unit of measure:

> Nearly three-fourths of my patients participate in a managed care plan.
>
> She came in to the office about an hour and a half later.

Type fractions using numbers when they are part of a compound modifier preceding a noun:

The abdomen shows a 4-1/4-inch scar.

5. There is often confusion with the phrase *pro time*, which is the shortened form of the laboratory term *prothrombin time*. Although some spell-check programs offer the option to replace the spelling error "protime" with "ProTime," this is incorrect. The expanded form of the word, *prothrombin time*, is preferred, but if the short form is used, it should be written as two words: *pro time*, not "protime."

> The patient's pro time was found to be elevated.

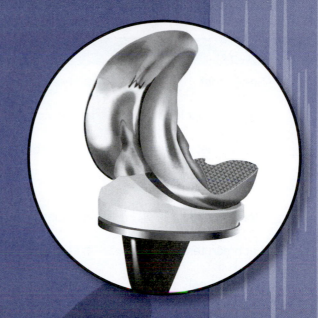

PROJECT 8

Orthopedics

TASK 8-1A: MATCHING EXERCISE

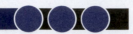

Instructions: Match the following common orthopedic muscle and flexibility tests in the left column with the corresponding part of the body for each test in the right column. Body parts can be used more than once.

Test	Body Part to be Tested
1. _____ Speed test	a. head
2. _____ manual muscle test	b. cervical spine
3. _____ Patrick test	c. shoulder
4. _____ Faber test	d. arm
5. _____ Romberg test	e. spine and/or hip
6. _____ Lachman test	f. leg
7. _____ Spurling test	g. muscle groups
8. _____ McMurray test	
9. _____ Finkelstein test	
10. _____ Tinel sign	
11. _____ Neer impingement test	
12. _____ cranial nerve exam	
13. _____ Murphy sign	
14. _____ Homans sign	
15. _____ Hawkins test	
16. _____ lift-off test	
17. _____ straight-leg raise	
18. _____ Phalen test	
19. _____ Apley scratch test	
20. _____ pivot shift test	

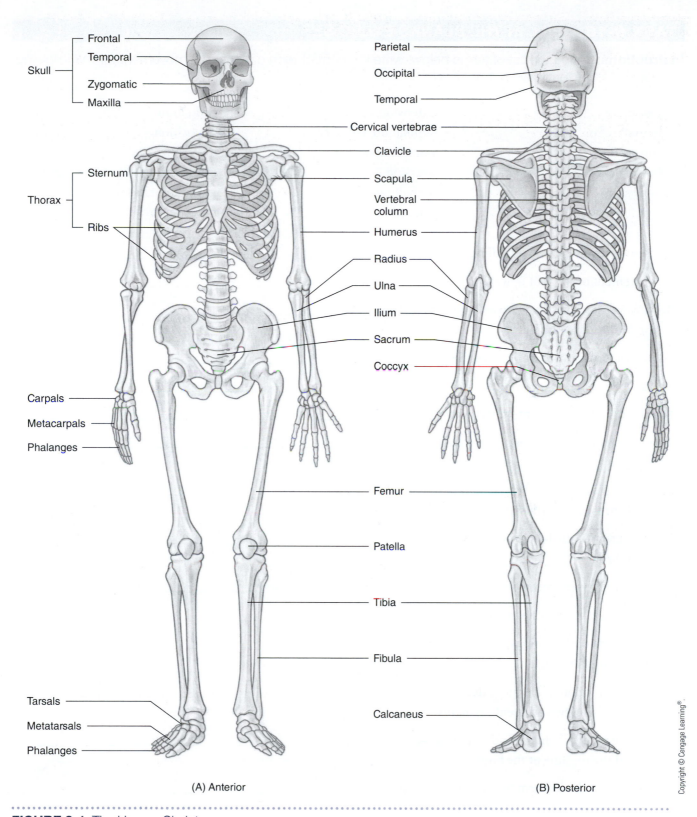

FIGURE 8-1 The Human Skeleton

TASK 8-1B: FILL IN THE BLANKS EXERCISE

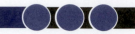

Instructions: Using the list of terms below, write the correct term of anatomic movement for the following definitions. Some terms will not be used.

flexion	extension	abduction
circumduction	supination	opposition
pronation	dorsiflexion	inversion
plantar flexion	eversion	external rotation
depression	adduction	internal rotation
elevation	retraction	protraction

1. To move away from the midline   _____

2. Movement of the foot upward toward the leg   _____

3. Movement of the foot outward so the outside of the foot is raised higher   _____

4. Rotation of the forearm to turn the palm down   _____

5. To move closer to the midline   _____

6. Moving a body part anteriorly   _____

7. Straightening motion of a joint to increase the angle between two adjacent segments   _____

8. Movement of the foot inward so the inside of the foot is raised higher   _____

9. Movement of the foot downward, away from the leg   _____

10. An upward movement   _____

11. Moving a body part posteriorly   _____

12. Movement of the hand where the thumb touches the fifth digit   _____

13. Bending motion of a joint to decrease the angle between two adjacent segments   _____

14. Movement of a joint around its long axis, toward the midline of the body   _____

15. Rotation of the forearm to turn the palm up   _____

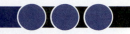

TASK 8-1C: MATCHING EXERCISE

Instructions: Match the following terms in the left column with the corresponding anatomic regions of the body in the right column.

Term	Anatomic Region
1. _____ cubital	A. armpit
2. _____ axillary	B. shoulder to elbow
3. _____ metacarpal	C. heel
4. _____ lumbar	D. neck
5. _____ nuchal	E. elbow
6. _____ plantar	F. great toe
7. _____ volar	G. lower back
8. _____ cervical	H. hand
9. _____ peroneal	I. foot
10. _____ tarsal	J. back of the neck
11. _____ popliteal	K. lower leg or fibula
12. _____ hallux	L. sole of the foot
13. _____ calcaneal	M. posterior knee
14. _____ brachial	N. ankle
15. _____ metatarsal	O. palm of the hand/sole of the foot

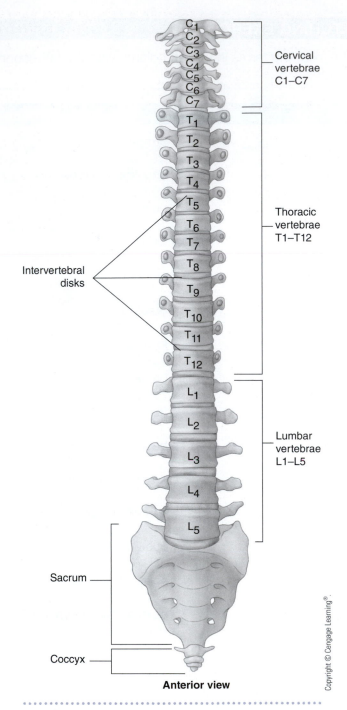

Cervical vertebrae C1–C7

Thoracic vertebrae T1–T12

Intervertebral disks

Lumbar vertebrae L1–L5

Sacrum

Coccyx

Anterior view

FIGURE 8-2 The Vertebral Column

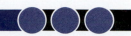

TASK 8-2:   PROOFREADING EXERCISES

Instructions: The proofreading documents below are designed to challenge your proofreading and editing skills. The documents may contain missing demographic information, incorrect headings, misspelled words, misplaced punctuation, and other errors within the document. Read each report below and identify the error by circling the word. Then retype the document with the corrected text and formatting. When finished, proofread your work and save the document to your student disk using a different file name.

PROOFREADING EXERCISE 1

PRIMARY DISCHARGE DIAGNOSIS: Right acromioclavicular seperation.

PROCEDURES: Open reduction internal fixation right acromioclavicular joint.

HISTORY: This is a 33-year-old who presented with pain in the right shoulder after a fall from a horse. X-rays revealed AC separation requiring open reduction and external fixation.

HOSPITAL COURSE: The patient was admitted and taken to the operating room for the abovenoted procedure. The postoperative course was uneventful, receiving 2 days of postoperative Kefzol and wearing a shoulder imobilizer.

DISPOSITION: The plan is for discharge to home, in good condition.

DISCHARGE MEDICATIONS:

1. Tylenol number 3, #30.
2. Ibuprofen 800 t.i.d., #60.
3. Dicloxacillin 500 q.i.d. for seven days.

ACTIVITY INSTRUCTIONS: Left shoulder immobilizer 24 hours a day and follow up in 3 days in the office.

PROOFREADING EXERCISE 2

DISCHARGE DIAGNOSIS:

1. Removal of hardware from left tibia status post open reduction and internal fixation 4 to 5 years ago.
2. Postoperative right lower lobe pneumonia with postoperative fever.
3. History of hypothyroidism.

HISTORY: A 52-year-old Latina female with pain in her left tibium since orif 5 years ago, admitted now for removal of hardware.

HOSPITAL COURSE: The plate and screws was removed without complications. She did well however postoperatively she developed fever, cough with sputum, and rhals in the left lower lobe. Chest x-ray demonstrated a small infiltrate. She was treated with Cefzol and improved with subsequent plan for discharge to home.

(Continues)

PROOFREADING EXERCISE 1 *(Continued)*

DISCHARGE MEDICATIONS:

1. Erythromycin 500 q.i.d. for 10 days.
2. Tylenol No. 3#30, no refills, to be taken as needed.
3. Ibuprofen 800 t.i.d., #60, no refills.
4. Continue thyroid medications as on admission.

DISCHARGE INSTRUCTIONS: He is to be non-weightbearing on crutches and follow up in 4 days in the office.

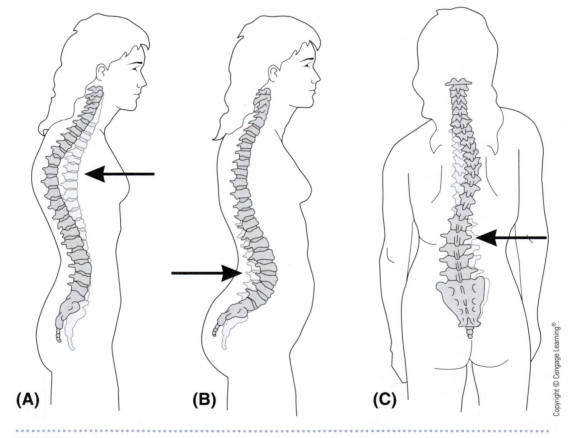

(A)   (B)   (C)

Copyright © Cengage Learning®.

FIGURE 8-3 Abnormal Curvature of the Spine: (A) Kyphosis, (B) Lordosis, (C) Scoliosis

ORTHOPEDICS TRANSCRIPTION TIPS

1. The terms *vagus* and *valgus* are often confused. *Vagus* refers to the nerve that travels through the body and supplies nerve signals to the pharynx, larynx, lungs, heart, esophagus, stomach, and most of the abdominal organs. *Valgus* refers to a deformity involving the bending or twisting away of a structure from the midline of the body.

2. Physicians will use the word *crepitations* to describe the noise produced when bone or irregular cartilage surfaces meet or rub together, such as in arthritis. Correct forms of the word are *crepitation*, *crepitus*, or *crepitant* (the adjective form), but not "creptitants" or "crepitance," as is often dictated.

3. Do not confuse the terms *metacarpal* and *metatarsal*. *Metacarpal* refers to the bones of the hand, whereas *metatarsal* refers to the bones of the foot.

4. Physicians refer to many specific orthopedic tests when examining a patient. If you cannot locate the name of the test in a medical dictionary or word book, try searching under the headings "test," "sign," or "maneuver" for the specific name of the test.

5. Remember that the muscles *biceps*, *triceps*, and *quadriceps* are always spelled the same in the singular and plural forms.

   The patient was diagnosed with a torn quadriceps femoris muscle.

   X-ray examination revealed a torn biceps tendon.

   During the fall, she injured both biceps muscles.

TASK 8-3: CLOZE EXERCISES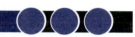

Instructions: The audio files for the following cloze exercises are located on the Premium website that accompanies this text (ISBN-13: 978-1-285-73537-5) at http://www.CengageBrain.com. If this is the first time you are registering your account, see the Preface for further instructions.

Once you are logged in to your account, locate the dictation file and Word document for the following cloze exercises. Open the audio file to be reviewed according to the exercise number indicated, along with its corresponding Word document. Listen to the dictation and read along with the text, filling in the missing words in the report by thinking critically and analytically about the context of the text you are reading. When finished, proofread your work and save the document according to your instructor's directions.

CLOZE EXERCISE 1: Lumbar MRI_Report 8
Patient Name: Cheryl Snyder
Medical Record Number: 94035

CLOZE EXERCISE 2: SOAP Note_Report 22
Patient Name: Sharon Norris
Medical Record Number: 25702

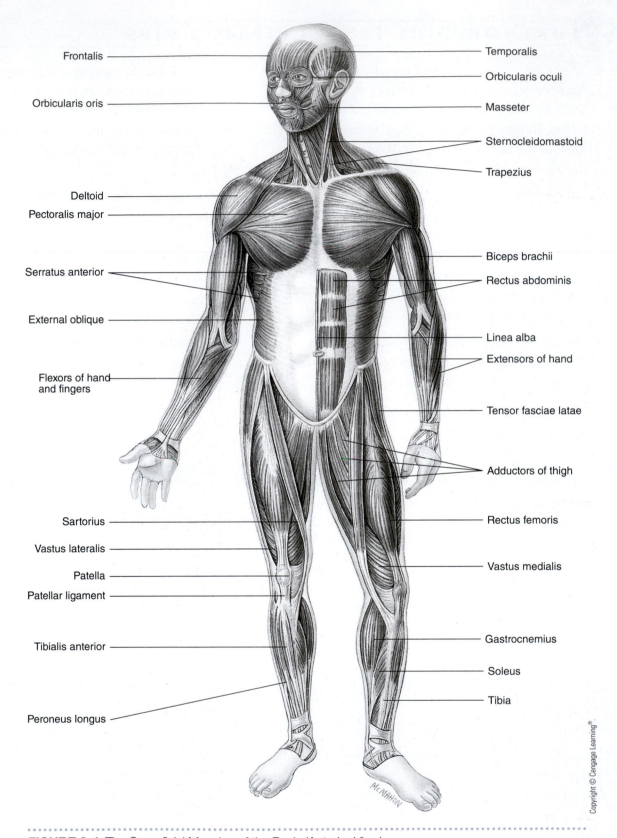

Frontalis

Orbicularis oris

Deltoid

Pectoralis major

Serratus anterior

External oblique

Flexors of hand and fingers

Sartorius

Vastus lateralis

Patella

Patellar ligament

Tibialis anterior

Peroneus longus

Temporalis

Orbicularis oculi

Masseter

Sternocleidomastoid

Trapezius

Biceps brachii

Rectus abdominis

Linea alba

Extensors of hand

Tensor fasciae latae

Adductors of thigh

Rectus femoris

Vastus medialis

Gastrocnemius

Soleus

Tibia

McMAHON

FIGURE 8-4 The Superficial Muscles of the Body (Anterior View)

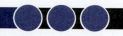

TASK 8-4: TRANSCRIPTION EXERCISES

Instructions: The audio files for the following transcription exercises are located on the Premium website that accompanies this text (ISBN-13: 978-1-285-73537-5) at http://www.CengageBrain.com. If this is the first time you are registering your account, see the Preface for further instructions.

Once you are logged in to your account, locate and open the audio file to be transcribed according to the exercise number indicated and transcribe each report. Do not insert a heading into the document if the text requires a second page, but let the text wrap naturally to the second page and continue typing. Transcribe the reports using the formatting specifics indicated in the Document Formatting Guidelines located at the beginning of this book. When finished, proofread your work and save the document according to your instructor's directions.

TRANSCRIPTION EXERCISE 1: Consultation_Report 1
Patient Name: Ernesto Flores
Medical Record Number: 06412

TRANSCRIPTION EXERCISE 2: Clinic Note_Report 8
Patient Name: Kathy Palmer
Medical Record Number: 11699

TRANSCRIPTION EXERCISE 3: MRI_Report 10
Patient Name: Damon Green
Medical Record Number: 94836

TRANSCRIPTION EXERCISE 4: SOAP Note_Report 7
Patient Name: Keisha Omehia
Medical Record Number: 43422

TRANSCRIPTION EXERCISE 5: Preoperative History and Physical_Report 13
Patient Name: Jake Rizzo
Medical Record Number: 98667

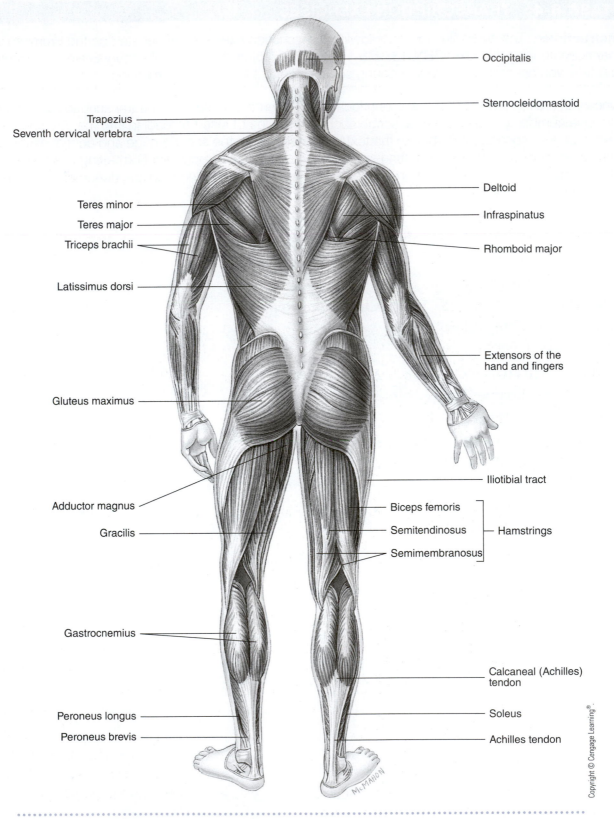

- Occipitalis
- Sternocleidomastoid
- Trapezius
- Seventh cervical vertebra
- Deltoid
- Infraspinatus
- Teres minor
- Teres major
- Triceps brachii
- Rhomboid major
- Latissimus dorsi
- Extensors of the hand and fingers
- Gluteus maximus
- Iliotibial tract
- Adductor magnus
- Biceps femoris
- Gracilis
- Semitendinosus
- Semimembranosus
- Hamstrings
- Gastrocnemius
- Calcaneal (Achilles) tendon
- Peroneus longus
- Soleus
- Peroneus brevis
- Achilles tendon

FIGURE 8-4 The Superficial Muscles of the Body (Posterior View)

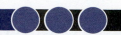

TASK 8-5: SPEECH RECOGNITION EXERCISES

Instructions: The audio files for the following speech recognition exercises are located on the Premium website that accompanies this text (ISBN-13: 978-1-285-73537-5) at http://www.CengageBrain.com. If this is the first time you are registering your account, see the Preface for further instructions.

Once you are logged in to your account, locate the dictation file and Word document for the following speech recognition exercises. Open the audio file to be reviewed according to the exercise number indicated, along with its corresponding Word document. Listen to the dictation and read along with the text, making corrections to the text with regard to formatting, terminology, grammar, spelling, and punctuation. When finished, proofread your work and save the document according to your instructor's directions.

SRT EXERCISE 1: Bone Scan_Report 12
Patient Name: Yuan Fong
Medical Record Number: 58226

SRT EXERCISE 2: Discharge Summary_Report 5
Patient Name: Drew Murphy
Medical Record Number: 54253

SRT EXERCISE 3: Discharge Summary_Report 6
Patient Name: Mary Grissom
Medical Record Number: 49211

SRT EXERCISE 4: Clinic Note_Report 7
Patient Name: Molly Redwood
Medical Record Number: 33740

COMPUTER SOFTWARE TIPS

1. To clear all the formatting in a document and return it to the default settings, first select the text to clear the formatting from. Then on the **Home** ribbon, click the **Clear Formatting** button located in the **Font** group, which looks like a piece of paper above a white eraser.

2. Check the **Check Grammar** box at the bottom of the **Spellcheck** dialog box to check both spelling and grammar in your document at the same time.

3. The **Research** button located in the **Proofing** group on the **Review Tab** opens the Research task pane with several reference options and online resources already selected for selected text.

4. You can enable Word to automatically hyphenate words in a document by selecting the **Page Layout** tab, then **Page Setup**, and clicking on **Automatic** in the **Hyphenation Gallery**.

5. If you want to add a border line in your document (such as beneath a header or above a footer), on the **Home** tab, choose the **Borders** drop-down box, then **Borders and Shading**, to make your selections.

ORTHOPEDICS BOOK OF STYLE TIPS

1. Use the spelling *disk* for all anatomic terms (including disks of the spine) other than ophthalmologic use, which uses *disc* (as in *optic disc*).

   optic disc

   L4-5 disk space

   diskectomy

   diskitis

2. When transcribing vertebrae of the spine:
   A. Type individual vertebrae without a hyphen.

      C1

      T2

   B. Type portions of a vertebra without a hyphen.

      C3 spinous process

      L4 lamina

      transverse process of T10

   C. Type a hyphen to express the space between two vertebrae.

      C1-2, or C1-C2

      L5-S1

   D. When expressing a range between two nonadjacent vertebrae where the word "through," not "to," is used, spell out and do not hyphenate.

      Dictated: We performed a fusion of T10 through T12.

      Transcribed: We performed a fusion of T10 through T12.

      not

      We performed a fusion of T10-T12.

      Rationale: To type T10-T12 would imply that T10 was fused to T12 rather than a procedure that involved fusion of T10 to T11, and T11 to T12.

3. Some specific terms heard in orthopedics include:
   A. *Weightbearing* (one word) and *weight bear* (two words).

      The patient was given instructions about weightbearing.

      The patient was told not to weight bear on her left leg for a week.

   B. *Fingerbreadth*, which refers to a unit of measure associated with the measurement by the hand of distance during a physical examination.

      The liver measured 3 fingerbreadths below the right costal margin.

   C. *Fluctuation* and *fluctuance*, which are synonymous noun forms of the word, not "fluctuants," which is not a word. The adjective form of the word is *fluctuant*.

      There is mild inflammation around the left lower anterior chest wound from the prior chest tube. However, there is no fluctuance.

   D. *Plane,* which describes an imaginary flat surface to provide anatomic orientation of the body. For example, the *frontal plane* divides the body into anterior and posterior sections. The *sagittal plane* divides the body into right and left sides. The *transverse plane* divides the body into upper and lower sections. The word "plain" refers to a type of radiographic image taken without the use of contrast dye or other materials.

4. Do not capitalize the words *sign*, *test*, or *score* even when they are associated with eponyms.

      Phalen sign

      drawer test

      Harris hip score

5. Type angles in orthopedic testing by writing out *degrees*, or you may use the degree sign if approved by your facility.

      The patient performed a straight-leg test to 50 degrees.

      The patient was able to straight leg raise to 50°.

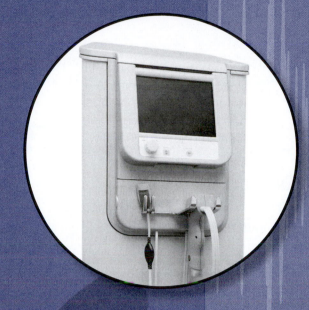

PROJECT 9

Dermatology

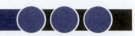

TASK 9-1A: FILL IN THE BLANKS EXERCISE

Instructions: Read the following clinic note and fill in the blanks in the record with the terms listed, relying on the context provided by the sentence to make your choices. Each term should be used only once.

sinus	CBC	graft
Staphylococcus	tract	dressing
plastic surgeon	osteomyelitis	Kerlix
culture	Hickman	aureus
humerus	saline	spinal

ADMISSION DIAGNOSIS: Chronic draining wounds of the left hip and left elbow.

DISCHARGE DIAGNOSES: Chronic draining wounds of the left elbow and left femur with methicillin-resistant Staphylococcus _____, status post muscle flap and skin graft to the hip, status post incision and drainage of the adjoining left elbow wound, urinary _____ infection, Pseudomonas, and development of a methicillin-resistant *Staphylococcus aureus* of the left elbow after treatment with medically resistant methicillin-resistant *Staphylococcus aureus* to the left hip.

HISTORY: The patient is a 42-year-old male with a history of quadriplegia following a C7 _____ injury years ago. The patient has been having a lot of trouble with some of his wounds and outpatient treatment was attempted with intravenous antibiotics through a _____ catheter. The patient was previously on vancomycin for an MRSA infection of the blood. Eventually, the cultures were negative; however, the patient has had increased drainage from the left hip and left elbow despite twice daily _____ changes. The patient also developed symptoms of fever and night sweats.

PHYSICAL EXAMINATION: On admission, the patient's temperature is 100.1 and he is in moderate distress. Examination of the patient's extremities shows a draining _____ of the upper right elbow with a purulent green discharge which was cultured. The left hip had similar discharge.

HOSPITAL COURSE: The patient was admitted and started on gentamicin. The wound _____ of the left elbow grew out *Staphylococcus aureus* and pseudomonas. His hip grew out MRSA. He was then changed to vancomycin. A _____ was consulted for a skin graft of the hip. After wound cultures were negative and following 3 weeks of IV vancomycin therapy, a skin _____ was attempted and performed.

Meanwhile, dressings were done on the left elbow and for the hip flap. When the dressings were taken off the left elbow, there was a question of whether there was early _____ on the distal posterior _____. The patient was scheduled for incision and drainage of the left elbow and eventually grew out pseudomonas

(Continues)

HOSPITAL COURSE: (Continued)

from his urine, and this was treated with Cipro. The left elbow was eventually grafted. The patient was deemed ready for discharge, when the cultures from the left elbow skin graft came back with methicillin-resistant _____ aureus again. The patient was started on vancomycin again. The patient was disappointed that he could not be discharged. He was treated with vancomycin for another 10 days and then discharged. Prior to discharge, the patient had been afebrile and off antibiotics for several days.

LABORATORY DATA: A _____ was checked prior to discharge and showed a WBC of 8700.

DISCHARGE INSTRUCTIONS: The patient will be followed up in 1 week. He must have dry dressings with dry gauze and _____ to the right elbow because this has been showing some skin breakdown. In addition, the patient is to clean the left elbow with normal _____ dressings on a daily basis and then apply a dry dressing. The patient is to return to the emergency room for any increased drainage, erythema, fever, chills, nausea, or vomiting.

DISCHARGE MEDICATIONS:

1. Vicodin 1 tablet p.o. q.4 h p.r.n.
2. Ditropan 10 mg p.o. b.i.d.
3. Meprobamate 100 mg p.o. q.i.d.

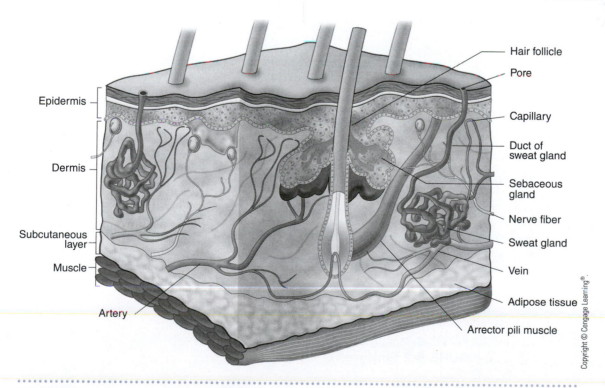

Epidermis

Dermis

Subcutaneous layer

Muscle

Artery

Hair follicle

Pore

Capillary

Duct of sweat gland

Sebaceous gland

Nerve fiber

Sweat gland

Vein

Adipose tissue

Arrector pili muscle

Copyright © Cengage Learning®.

FIGURE 9-1 The Structures of the Skin

TASK 9-1B: MEDICAL WORD BUILDING EXERCISE

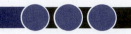

Instructions: From the list given, write the correct surgical term next to each phrase or characteristic indicated.

dermabrasion

excision

suturing

incision and drainage

cauterization

debridement

Mohs surgery

incision

cryosurgery

laser surgery

1. use of electric current   _____

2. use of extreme cold   _____

3. uses a high-powered beam of light   _____

4. removal with abrasive materials, like sandpaper   _____

5. closing the edges of a wound surgically   _____

6. to remove by cutting   _____

7. to cut into a wound with a sharp instrument   _____

8. removal of dead or damaged tissue from a wound   _____

9. microscopically controlled removal of skin cancers   _____

10. a cut into a wound to allow the removal of fluid from a wound   _____

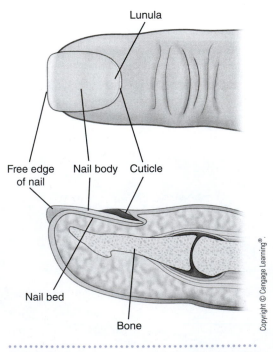

FIGURE 9-2 Structures of the Fingernails and Toenails

TASK 9-1C: MULTIPLE CHOICE EXERCISE

Instructions: Choose the correct abbreviations to complete the following sentences.

1. One symptom of _____ is a red rash on the cheeks of the face.
   - **A.** DLE
   - **B.** BCC
   - **C.** CMV
   - **D.** SLE

2. The combination of psoralen and ultraviolet light applied to the skin is known as _____ therapy.
   - **A.** UVA
   - **B.** PUVA
   - **C.** PCOM
   - **D.** HBOT

3. The _____ test is named after the chemical formula for potassium hydroxide.
   - **A.** KOH
   - **B.** BCC
   - **C.** NIH
   - **D.** TD

4. _____ is the most common complication of herpes zoster, which is chronic pain in the area of a shingles outbreak.
   - **A.** PCH
   - **B.** NIH
   - **C.** PNH
   - **D.** ID

5. A class of drugs called _____, which include drugs such as Elidel and Protopic, has been developed for use in severe cases of eczema.
   - **A.** METs
   - **B.** TIMs
   - **C.** BOTs
   - **D.** TBs

6. _____ light alters the chemicals in skin cells and can kill certain cells that can be involved in skin disease.
   - **A.** PUV
   - **B.** UX
   - **C.** UV
   - **D.** XR

7. The patient visited the _____ clinic for a followup visit of her cystitis.
   - **A.** GU
   - **B.** OB
   - **C.** GI
   - **D.** GYN

8. _____ is the most common form of skin cancer and accounts for more than 90% of all skin cancers in the United States.
   - **A.** SqCCA
   - **B.** PSA
   - **C.** BC
   - **D.** BCC

9. A _____ of the lesion was taken and was found to be negative.
   A. DX
   B. BX
   C. MX
   D. BB

10. One of the yeast organisms that cause skin infection in humans is called _____ *albicans.*
   A. *A.*
   B. *D.*
   C. *C.*
   D. *S.*

TASK 9-2: PROOFREADING EXERCISES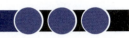

Instructions: The proofreading documents below are designed to challenge your proofreading and editing skills. The documents may contain missing demographic information, incorrect headings, misspelled words, misplaced punctuation, and other errors within the document. Read each report below and identify the error by circling the word. Then retype the document with the corrected text and formatting. When finished, proofread your work and save the document to your student disk using a different file name.

PROOFREADING EXERCISE 1

ADMISSION DIAGNOSES: Sacral decubitus ulcer.

SECONDARY DIAGNOSES: Severe dementia, probable presenting Alzheimer's disease, severe generalized wasting with poor nutrition and flexion contractions, and probable congestive heart failure with pneumonia.

PROCEDURE: Debridement of infected sacral decubitus ulcer.

HISTORY: This is a 98 year old woman who was brought to the hospital from a local nursing home for surgical debridement of a deep infected decubitus ulcer. The patients condition has been poor. She is profoundly demented and is essentially in a vegetative state on admission.

PHYSICAL EXAMINATION: The physical examination revealed an obviously bedridden, demented patient with flexion contractures, a deep decubitus ulcer of the sacral area, secondarily infected.

LABORATORY DATA: White count was 15.6, increased to 20,300, with 92% neutrophil and 1 percent bands. The hemoglobin initially was 15.4 and then dropped to 12.8. Bun was 21 on admission, creatinine 0.8, total protein 5.5 and albumin 2.0.

Urinanalysis showed marked pyuria on avoided specimen.

Blood culture showed no growth. The urine culture was positive for proteus mirabilisvand sputum culture is pending.

The EKG was abnormal, showing atrial fibrillation and nonspecific STT abnormalities. Chest X-ray was abnormal, showing evidence of congestive failure and possible pneumonia at left lung base.

(Continues)

PROOFREADING EXERCISE 1 *(Continued)*

HOSPITAL COURSE: The patient's wound was debrided under local anesthesia, treated with diuretics and intervenous antibiotics until she was stable. She was then transferred back to the nursing home. Because of her poor condition overall, the patient's sun requested she not be treated with antibiotics or any lifesustaining treatment. These orders for the extent of treatment were to be carried over to the Nursing Home.

PROOFREADING EXERCISE 2

DISCHARGE DIAGNOSES:

1. Pylonidal cyst with right buttocks abscess, resolving.
2. Diabetes mellitus with the patient started on sulfurnylurea.
3. Hypertension, stable.
4. Alcohol abuse.

PROCEDURE PERFORMED: Incision and drainage of right buttock absess.

BRIEF HISTORY: The patient was admitted to the surgical service for treatment. The patient had his wound incisioned and drained on the first hospital day, with bloody exudate being obtained. The patient was on intraveneous antibiotics throughout his hospital course and had BID dressing changes. He had slow resolution of his abscess. Otherwise, the patient was feeling well. The patient was discharged home on hospital day no. 5. On discharge the patient was afebrile and with stable vital signs he was eating and ambulating well. His nephew was instructed in dressing change techniques and he feels comfortable with this. She was observed by the nursing staff to do a good job prior to the patient's discharge.

LABORATORY DATA: The culture from the emergency room aspirate was negative after 48 hours.

DISCHARGE MEDICATIONS:

1. Dicloxacillin 500 mg PO q.i.d.
2. Tylenol #3 one tablet p.o. q 4 hours p.r.n. pain.

DISCHARGE PLANS:

1. The patient is to followup in 1 week in the office.
2. He will have b.i.d. dressing changes and sits baths at home.

DERMATOLOGY TRANSCRIPTION **TIPS**

1. Drug reactions and viral skin lesions may be described as *maculopapular*, consisting of both *macules* and *papules*. Do not transcribe this description as "macular papular."

2. Burns can be *partial-thickness* or *full-thickness* injuries. Do not transcribe this as "partial-sickness" or "full-sickness."

3. Some dictators may assess a skin lesion using the acronym *ABCDE* to describe a lesion's characteristics, which means **a**symmetry, **b**order irregularity, **c**olor variation, **d**iameter of more than 6 mm, and **e**volutionary change of the lesion.

4. *Mohs microscopic surgery* was named after its inventor, Dr. Frederick Mohs. Do not add an apostrophe to the name ("Moh's") when typing reports that refer to *Mohs surgery*, as this is incorrect.

5. Be careful to distinguish the soundalike words *bullous*, which relates to a *bulla*, or a fluid-filled blister or bubblelike structure on the skin, and *bolus*, which is a single dosage of a substance intended for therapeutic use, such as in a dose of a drug.

TASK 9-3: CLOZE EXERCISES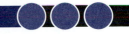

Instructions: The audio files for the following cloze exercises are located on the Premium website that accompanies this text (ISBN-13: 978-1-285-73537-5) at http://www.CengageBrain.com. If this is the first time you are registering your account, see the Preface for further instructions.

Once you are logged in to your account, locate the dictation file and Word document for the following cloze exercises. Open the audio file to be reviewed according to the exercise number indicated, along with its corresponding Word document. Listen to the dictation and read along with the text, filling in the missing words in the report by thinking critically and analytically about the context of the text you are reading. When finished, proofread your work and save the document according to your instructor's directions.

CLOZE EXERCISE 1: SOAP Note_Report 5
Patient Name: Kim Hoffman
Medical Record Number: 88492

CLOZE EXERCISE 2: Clinic Note_Report 17
Patient Name: Deborah Elliott
Medical Record Number: 88748

TASK 9-4: TRANSCRIPTION EXERCISES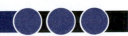

Instructions: The audio files for the following transcription exercises are located on the Premium website that accompanies this text (ISBN-13: 978-1-285-73537-5) at http://www.CengageBrain.com. If this is the first time you are registering your account, see the Preface for further instructions.

Once you are logged in to your account, locate and open the audio file to be transcribed according to the exercise number indicated and transcribe each report. Do not insert a heading into the document if the text requires a second page, but let the text wrap naturally to the second page and continue typing. Transcribe the reports using the formatting specifics indicated in the Document Formatting Guidelines located at the beginning of this book. When finished, proofread your work and save the document according to your instructor's directions.

TRANSCRIPTION EXERCISE 1: Operative Note_Report 14
Patient Name: Michael Jones
Medical Record Number: 19758

TRANSCRIPTION EXERCISE 2: Discharge Summary_Report 11
Patient Name: William Collins96951
Medical Record Number: 37078

TRANSCRIPTION EXERCISE 3: Procedure Note_Report 4
Patient Name: Benjamin Robinson
Medical Record Number: 18701

TRANSCRIPTION EXERCISE 4: Discharge Summary_Report 2
Patient Name: Helen Kelly
Medical Record Number: 01125

TRANSCRIPTION EXERCISE 5: History and Physical_Report 12
Patient Name: Myron Lewis
Medical Record Number: 27561

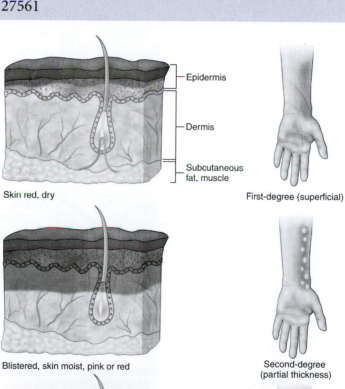
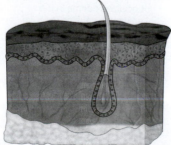
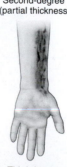

Epidermis

Dermis

Subcutaneous fat, muscle

Skin red, dry

First-degree (superficial)

Blistered, skin moist, pink or red

Second-degree (partial thickness)

Charring, skin black, brown, red

Third-degree (full thickness)

FIGURE 9-3 The Degree of Burn as Determined by the Length of Skin Involved

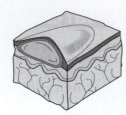

Bulla: (Large blister)
Same as a vesicle only greater than 10 mm
Example:
Contact dermatitis, large second degree burns, bulbous impetigo, pemphigus

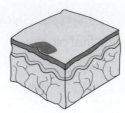

Macule:
Localized changes in skin color of less than 1 cm in diameter
Example:
Freckle

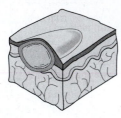

Nodules:
Solid and elevated; however, they extend deeper than papules into the dermis or subcutaneous tissues, greater than 10 mm
Example:
Lipoma, erythema, cyst, wart

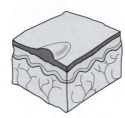

Papule:
Solid, elevated lesion less than 1 cm in diameter
Example:
Elevated nevi

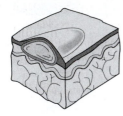

Pustule:
Vesicles or bullae that become filled with pus, usually described as less than 0.5 cm in diameter
Example:
Acne, impetigo, furuncles, carbuncles

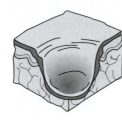

Ulcer:
A depressed lesion of the epidermis and upper papillary layer of the dermis
Example:
Stage 2 pressure ulcer

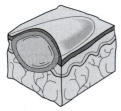

Tumor:
The same as a nodule only greater than 2 cm

Example:
Benign epidermal tumor basal cell carcinoma

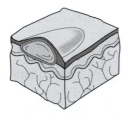

Vesicle: (Small blister)
Accumulation of fluid between the upper layers of the skin; elevated mass containing serous fluid; less than 10 mm
Example:
Herpes simplex, herpes zoster, chickenpox

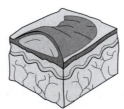

Urticaria, Hives:
Localized edema in the epidermis causing irregular elevation that may be red or pale, may be itchy
Example:
Insect bite, wheal

FIGURE 9-4 Different Types of Skin Lesions

TASK 9-5: SPEECH RECOGNITION EXERCISES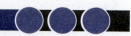

Instructions: The audio files for the following speech recognition exercises are located on the Premium website that accompanies this text (ISBN-13: 978-1-285-73537-5) at http://www.CengageBrain.com. If this is the first time you are registering your account, see the Preface for further instructions.

Once you are logged in to your account, locate the dictation file and Word document for the following speech recognition exercises. Open the audio file to be reviewed according to the exercise number indicated, along with its corresponding Word document. Listen to the dictation and read along with the text, making corrections to the text with regard to formatting, terminology, grammar, spelling, and punctuation. When finished, proofread your work and save the document according to your instructor's directions.

SRT EXERCISE 1: SOAP Note_Report 4
Patient Name: Sandy Dunn
Medical Record Number: 14471

SRT EXERCISE 2: Discharge Summary_Report 10
Patient Name: Teresa Herrera
Medical Record Number: 13814

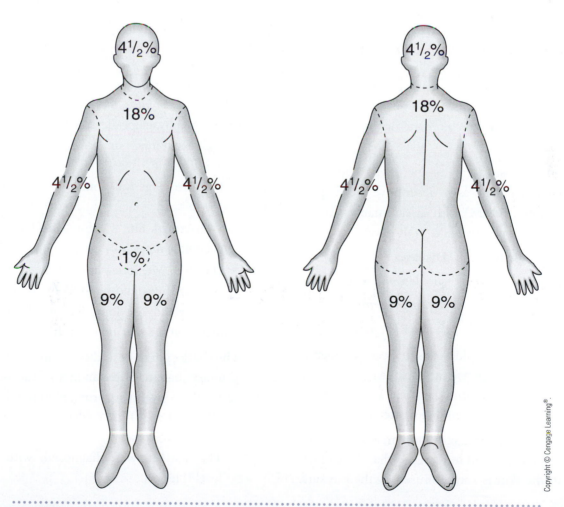

FIGURE 9-5 The Rule of Nines Diagram Used to Calculate the Percentage of Body Surface Burned, Which Divides the Body into 11 Areas with Each Area Accounting for 9% of the Total Body Surface

COMPUTER SOFTWARE **TIPS**

1. Use **CTRL + S** to save a document instead of navigating the Office button with the mouse.

2. If you want to see the gridlines in a table you have created, select the table and on the **Layout** Ribbon, select the **Show Gridlines** option located in the **Table** group.

3. Comments are little notes you can add to a document without disturbing its content. The comment appears in the right margin in a box with your initials. To add a comment, highlight the area of the document you want to comment on and on the Reviewing tab, press the New Comment button. Then type your comment text in the box that appears.

4. You can add an envelope to print along with a letter in the same document. On the Ribbon, open the **Mailings** tab, click the **Envelopes** button, type the envelope information in the boxes provided, and then click **Add to Document** to add the envelope to the letter in the Word document screen.

5. You can use either the F2 function key or **CTRL + X** to quickly cut text from a document to paste elsewhere. If the F2 function key is used, a query will appear in the lower left corner of the status bar prompting you to move your cursor to the new location.

DERMATOLOGY BOOK OF STYLE **TIPS**

1. *Naris* is the term given to one nostril of the nose; the plural term is *nares*. Physicians sometimes erroneously dictate this as "nare" or "naree," which is incorrect.

2. Do not confuse dermatologic terms ending in *-form* (which denotes a descriptive word, pronounced like FORM) with disease names ending in *-forme*, (pronounced like FOR-may).

Dermatologic terms	Diseases
herpetiform	*glioblastoma multiforme*
filiform	*urticaria multiforme*
acneiform	*Lycoperdon pyriforme*

3. Terms that describe skin tests to assess for allergic sensitivity and response can include *prick, scratch, challenge, patch,* or *RAST* testing. Except for the acronym, these test terms are written in lowercase.

4. A *decubitus ulcer* is a skin ulcer that comes from lying in one position too long so that the circulation in the skin is compromised by the pressure.

It is also known as a bed sore or pressure ulcer. The full term *decubitus ulcer* should be transcribed when the physician dictates either the shortened term, "decubitus," or erroneously dictates the plural "decubiti."

Dictated: She was found to have a stage II decubitus.

Transcribed: She was found to have a stage II decubitus ulcer.

Dictated: Mr. Jones has two deep decubiti on the sacrum extending to the ischium.

Transcribed: Mr. Jones has two deep decubitus ulcers on the sacrum extending to the ischium.

5. The Clark system describes the invasion level of a primary malignant melanoma of the skin. Transcribe these levels using roman numerals I (denoting the least deep) to IV (deepest), with the word "level" in lowercase.

The patient was diagnosed with a Clark level II lesion.

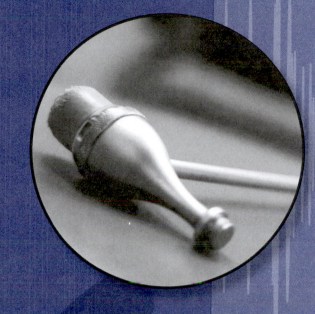

PROJECT 10

Neurology

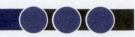

TASK 10-1A: MULTIPLE CHOICE EXERCISE

Instructions: Circle the letter corresponding to the best answer to each of the following questions.

1. There are _____ sets of spinal nerves, which come from the spinal cord and pass between vertebral pairs.
   A. 31
   B. 13
   C. 30
   D. 10

2. _____ is a sensory and motor disorder that occurs when cells in the central nervous system lose myelin, leading to the deterioration of nerve function.
   A. Myeloma
   B. Parkinson disease
   C. Multiple sclerosis
   D. Alzheimer dementia

3. A person with parkinsonism experiences a resting tremor in one extremity in addition to _____
   A. thrombocytopenia.
   B. bradykinesia.
   C. tachycardia.
   D. None of the above.

4. A transient ischemic attack (TIA) is often called a (an) _____
   A. seizure.
   B. sympathetic nervous system disorder.
   C. cranial nerve abnormality.
   D. mini-stroke.

5. Coordination of voluntary motor activities takes place in the _____
   A. cerebrum.
   B. cerebellum.
   C. brain stem.
   D. left frontal lobe.

6. The _____ contains the brain and the spinal cord.
   A. cerebellum
   B. peripheral nervous system
   C. central nervous system
   D. autonomic nervous system

7. The brain and spinal cord are covered by a protective layer of clear, colorless fluid called _____
   A. CSF.
   B. CNS.
   C. EEG.
   D. NCV.

8. A physician rotates a patient's head from side to side to observe the effect on eye position, called doll's eyes. Failure of the eyes to rotate around their own vertical axes indicates _____
   A. a high Glasgow coma score.
   B. hydrocephalus.
   C. disequilibrium.
   D. brain stem damage.

9. Impairment of proprioceptive impulses from the muscles of the limbs is called _____
   A. causalgia.
   B. paresthesia.
   C. ataxia.
   D. hemiplegia.

10. Another word for fainting is
    A. syncope.
    B. coma.
    C. paraplegia.
    D. none of the above.

11. _____ is the word that means "unable to speak."
    A. Dysphagia
    B. Aphasia
    C. Hyperphagia
    D. Aphakia

12. The optic nerve is also known as cranial nerve _____
    A. 2 (or II).
    B. 3 (or III).
    C. 4 (or IV).
    D. 5 (or V).

13. A type of test used to evaluate a patient's coordination and equilibrium is known as _____
    A. Wada.
    B. Prevnar.
    C. Romberg.
    D. Glasgow.

14. The Babinski test is performed on the _____
    A. hand.
    B. shoulder.
    C. knee.
    D. foot.

15. Another name for absence seizures is _____
    A. simple partial seizures.
    B. petit-mal seizures.
    C. myoclonic seizures.
    D. atonic seizures.

16. Pain that is produced by all stimuli to the skin that do not normally induce pain (such as touch or warmth) is called _____
    A. hyperesthesia.
    B. hyperpathia.
    C. allodynia.
    D. hyperhidrosis.

17. _____ is a painful condition caused by the herpes zoster virus that infects a nerve.
    A. Meningioma
    B. Varicella
    C. Shingles
    D. Cerebral palsy

18. Abnormal burning, prickling, or tingling sensations on the skin are called _____
    A. paresthesias.
    B. polyneuritis.
    C. paralysis.
    D. hemiplegia.

19. Which of the following is not a congenital neurologic disorder?
    A. Myelomeningocele
    B. Cerebral palsy
    C. Neurosarcoidosis
    D. None of the above

20. Which is not a symptom of migraine headaches?
    A. Photophobia
    B. Status epilepticus
    C. Throbbing pain
    D. Nausea

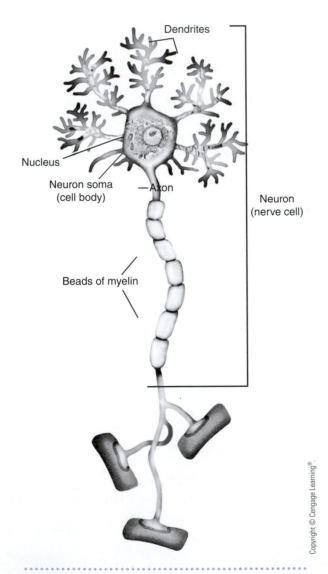

FIGURE 10-1 A Neuron is the Nerve Cell that Carries Out the Functions of the Central Nervous System

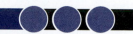

TASK 10-1B: MEDICAL COMPREHENSION EXERCISE

Instructions: Read the clinic note below and answer the questions that follow.

Today I had the pleasure of seeing Christina, a 9-month-old female, in Pediatric Neurosurgery Outpatient Clinic. This is the first time I have seen this little girl with her mother. According to the mother, she was in a department store shopping cart when she fell out of the cart and sustained a head injury. She did not lose consciousness and did not vomit. She cried immediately, and she was sent to Lutheran General Hospital emergency room where the acute care was done, and then she was admitted for observation. She was evaluated by the neurosurgeon. A CT scan apparently was obtained. Then she was discharged to home and she has been doing well, and Mom feels that she has never showed any symptoms such as vomiting, seizures, or lethargy, except she rubs her head from side to side.

Review of systems shows that there are no allergies, no vomiting, no seizures, and no lethargy. Eating habits are unchanged. No chest problems, no heart problems, abdomen is negative, and locomotor functions are age appropriate.

I reviewed the CT scan that was done at Lutheran General Hospital. This showed depressed fracture of the right parietal area about 4 to 5 mm in depth with questionable contusion but no intracranial hematoma.

Neurologic examination: She is alert and fully oriented. Anterior fontanel is soft and sunken. The right parietal area: One can palpate a slight depression in that area without any subgaleal hematoma. Pupils are 3 mm bilaterally. EOMs are full. There is no facial nerve paralysis. There is no tenderness over that depressed skull fracture area. No palpable mass, either. There is no motor weakness, without any lateralizing neurologic signs. DTRs are 2+ bilaterally. Babinski sign is negative.

It is my impression that she is status post depressed skull fracture of the right midparietal area and also with normal neurological findings. I discussed at length regarding the status of the depressed skull fracture and benign neurological finding without any focal lateralizing signs. I also reminded the mother to watch over her for any occurrence of seizures. Otherwise, I do not see any need of repeating CT scan at this time; however, as she progresses, I would consider repeating imaging of the brain, this time with MRI. Otherwise, I would like to see the child again in 4 months at the outpatient clinic. All the questions were answered for her.

1. When the Babinski sign is negative, it means that _____
   A. toes are upgoing.
   B. toes are downgoing.

2. What symptoms did the mother look for to indicate brain damage? _____
   _____ _____

3. The patient's eye movements were described as being _____
   A. paralyzed.
   B. full.
   C. soft and sunken.

4. Was the CT scan normal?
   A. Yes
   B. No

5. The physician's exam indicated that the deep tendon reflexes were _____
   A. hyperreflexive.
   B. normal.
   C. trace.
   D. absent.

6. What was the plan for the patient?
   A. To "watch and wait" and then return
   B. Admit the child immediately
   C. Repeat the CT scan next week
   D. Release the patient from the doctor's care

7. The doctor found the patient to be _____
   A. lethargic.
   B. nauseated.
   C. crying excessively.
   D. fully cognitive.

8. Which fontanel did the doctor comment on?
   A. The one in the back
   B. The one on the right side
   C. The one in the front
   D. None of them

9. What specifically was mentioned that the doctor did *not* find on review of the scan and his examination?
   A. A skull fracture
   B. Perhaps a bruise
   C. A depressed area
   D. A mass of clotted blood

10. Did the child have difficulty moving her arms and legs after the accident?
    A. Yes
    B. No

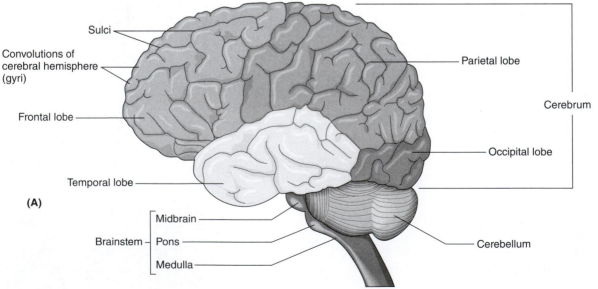

FIGURE 10-2 (A) The Major Parts of the Brain and (B) Areas of Brain Function

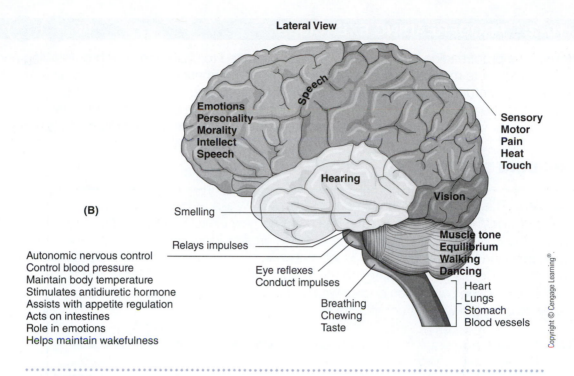

Lateral View

Emotions
Personality
Morality
Intellect
Speech

Speech

Sensory
Motor
Pain
Heat
Touch

Hearing

Vision

(B)

Smelling

Muscle tone
Equilibrium
Walking
Dancing

Autonomic nervous control
Control blood pressure
Maintain body temperature
Stimulates antidiuretic hormone
Assists with appetite regulation
Acts on intestines
Role in emotions
Helps maintain wakefulness

Relays impulses

Eye reflexes
Conduct impulses

Breathing
Chewing
Taste

Heart
Lungs
Stomach
Blood vessels

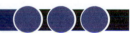

FIGURE 10-2 (*Continued*)

TASK 10-1C: MATCHING EXERCISE

Instructions: Match the term in the right column with its definition or description in the left column.

1. _____ regulates automatic functions		A. meninges
2. _____ a gland that helps the body produce hormones it needs to respond to various situations		B. CSF
		C. pituitary
3. _____ nerve cells		D. hypothalamus
4. _____ the watery substance that surrounds the brain		E. cerebrum
5. _____ protective connective tissue layers covering the brain		F. neurons
6. _____ the uppermost and largest part of the brain		G. ventricles
7. _____ the "thinking brain"		H. cerebellum
8. _____ the protective covering of the neuron		I. myelin sheath
9. _____ four small chambers connected to the spinal cord		J. cerebral cortex
10. _____ the "little brain" attached to the brainstem		

TASK 10-2: PROOFREADING EXERCISES

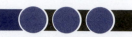

Instructions: The proofreading documents below are designed to challenge your proofreading and editing skills. The documents may contain missing demographic information, incorrect headings, misspelled words, misplaced punctuation, and other errors within the document. Read each report below and identify the error by circling the word. Then retype the document with the corrected text and formatting. When finished, proofread your work and save the document to your student disk using a different file name.

PROOFREADING EXERCISE 1

SUBJECTIVE: This 38-year-old female complains of 2 weeks of low back pain. She woke 1 morning with this discomfort. She has done no new exercise and has not had any injuries. She is overweight and does not exercise on a regular basis. She cares for several children and does lift two who weigh between 34-40 pounds. Patient states the pain is dull and constant. It radiates to the left buttock and leg occasionally, this is described as a shooting pain which occurs with certain movements. She is otherwise in her usual state of health without complaints.

OBJECTIVE: Muskuloskeletal: Back has full range of motion forward backward and sideward bending. No spinous process tenderness. There is paraspinal muscle tenderness with spasm noted in the low thoracic and upper lumber area. No skin changes are noted. Lower extremities have 5 over 5 muscle strength grossly, 2/4 patellar reflex. Negative slr.

ASSESSMENT/PLAN: Low back pain with muscle spasm. Skelaxin 400 mg 2 p.o. q6h. for 3 to 5 days, and Motrin 800 mg 1 p.o. q.8h. with food for 1 to 2 weeks, then p.r.n. No lifting greater than ten pounds for 1 week. Recommend bed rest on a firm surface. Patient given exercise sheet to be done after acute fase. Follow up on a p.r.n. bases.

PROOFREADING EXERCISE 2

HISTORY: Low back pane radiating into the right leg.

INTERPRETATION: The patient has a normal appearance of the conis medularis and the upper lumbar disk levels are well-maintained down to L2-L3. The L3,L4 area shows mild degenerative disc signal with only very slight narrowing. There is a small amount of posterior spurring at the L3-L4 innerspace, which combines with faset and ligamentus flavum hypertrophy to cause a mild degree of central spinal stenosis and lateral rescess narrowing.

The L45 area shows moderate narrowing and more vocal disk herniation that begins in the midline at the disk space and then just below the disk level extends eccentrically toward the right side. On the t1 axial images, we can see displacement and obscurity of the fat plain around the right L5 nerve root as it branches off, although the saggital images are not dramatic, I believe as they come over towards the right side that there is a disk herniation that is extending down over the lip of the L4-L5 interspace toward the right side. The L5-S11 area also shows moderate degenerative disk narrowing and a midline central disk protruding causing approximately a 3 mm extradural defect on the

(Continues)

PROOFREADING EXERCISE 2 *(Continued)*

thecal sack in the midline. This L5-S1 disk protrusion could be affecting the S1 or S2 roots as they begin to branch off, but I do not see any localization towards the right at this level. There are some degenerative facet disease at both L4-L5 and L5-S1, but no central spinal stenosis at these levels. The right L4-L5 formen is compromised by the posteriolateral disk herniation and facet change.

IMPRESSION: Mild degenerative disk changes at L3-L4 and a moderate degree of central spinal stenosis at this level, some posterior spurring and facet and ligamentum flavum changes. Focal disk herniation at the L4-L5 level that is ecentric toward the right side and extends a short way below the L-4-L-5 disk to elevate and obscure nerve roots around the right L5 rooot as it branches off. There is a mild right L4-L5 foraminal narrowing from the posterolateral disk protrusion and facet change, but no definite compermise of the right L4 root.

A central 3 mm disk protrusion at the L5-S1 level causing mild mass affect on the cecal sac and S1 roots as they branch off.

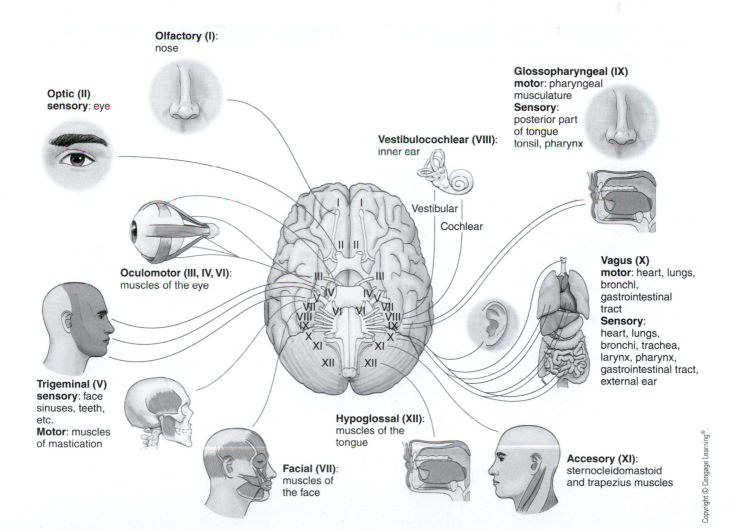

Olfactory (I):
nose

Optic (II)
sensory: eye

Glossopharyngeal (IX)
motor: pharyngeal musculature
Sensory: posterior part of tongue tonsil, pharynx

Vestibulocochlear (VIII):
inner ear

Vestibular
Cochlear

Oculomotor (III, IV, VI):
muscles of the eye

Vagus (X)
motor: heart, lungs, bronchi, gastrointestinal tract
Sensory: heart, lungs, bronchi, trachea, larynx, pharynx, gastrointestinal tract, external ear

Trigeminal (V)
sensory: face sinuses, teeth, etc.
Motor: muscles of mastication

Hypoglossal (XII):
muscles of the tongue

Facial (VII):
muscles of the face

Accesory (XI):
sternocleidomastoid and trapezius muscles

FIGURE 10-3 Cranial Nerve Function

NEUROLOGY TRANSCRIPTION TIPS

1. Do not confuse the abbreviations *CNS* and *C & S* when heard in dictation. *CNS* stands for central nervous system, while *C & S* means culture and sensitivity. Be sure to listen to the context of what is being said to choose the correct abbreviation.

2. In the neurologic exam, the dictator may state that a test is "equivocal," meaning that the results are not clear. Do not transcribe this as "equal."

3. Dictators may describe a "paucity of ideas" or "paucity of speech," meaning that the patient seems to have few ideas or limited speech. Do not mistranscribe this as *posity* or *aposity*.

4. When talking about aneurysms, physicians use the abbreviations *ACOM* (for anterior communicating artery) or *PCOM* (posterior communicating artery) and may say it like "A-COM" and "P-COM." Be sure to spell the terms correctly when transcribing them.

5. Be careful with the soundalike words *electroencephalogram (EEG)* and *electrocardiogram (EKG)*. An *EEG* is a test that measures and records the electrical activity of the brain. An *EKG* is a test that measures and records the electrical activity of the heart.

TASK 10-3: CLOZE EXERCISES

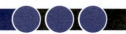

Instructions: The audio files for the following cloze exercises are located on the Premium website that accompanies this text (ISBN-13: 978-1-285-73537-5) at http://www.CengageBrain.com. If this is the first time you are registering your account, see the Preface for further instructions.

Once you are logged in to your account, locate the dictation file and Word document for the following cloze exercises. Open the audio file to be reviewed according to the exercise number indicated, along with its corresponding Word document. Listen to the dictation and read along with the text, filling in the missing words in the report by thinking critically and analytically about the context of the text you are reading. When finished, proofread your work and save the document according to your instructor's directions.

CLOZE EXERCISE 1: Clinic Note_Report 12
Patient Name: Melissa O'Brien
Medical Record Number: 44711

CLOZE EXERCISE 2: Clinic Note_Report 31
Patient Name: Laura Hart
Medical Record Number: 38810

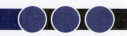

TASK 10-4: TRANSCRIPTION EXERCISES

Instructions: The audio files for the following transcription exercises are located on the Premium website that accompanies this text (ISBN-13: 978-1-285-73537-5) at http://www.CengageBrain.com. If this is the first time you are registering your account, see the Preface for further instructions.

Once you are logged in to your account, locate and open the audio file to be transcribed according to the exercise number indicated and transcribe each report. Do not insert a heading into the document if the text requires a second page, but let the text wrap naturally to the second page and continue typing. Transcribe the reports using the formatting specifics indicated in the Document Formatting Guidelines located at the beginning of this book. When finished, proofread your work and save the document according to your instructor's directions.

TRANSCRIPTION EXERCISE 1: Brain Scan_Report 9
Patient Name: Abdul Hasan
Medical Record Number: 41564

TRANSCRIPTION EXERCISE 2: Letter_Report 11
Patient Name: Marjorie Smith
Medical Record Number: 57826

TRANSCRIPTION EXERCISE 3: Clinic Note_Report 9027
Patient Name: Lauren Weller
Medical Record Number: 81747

TRANSCRIPTION EXERCISE 4: CT Scan of the Brain_Report 3102
Patient Name: Jose Ramos
Medical Record Number: 36277

TRANSCRIPTION EXERCISE 5: Clinic Note_Report 9031
Patient Name: Jennifer Bradley
Medical Record Number: 73688

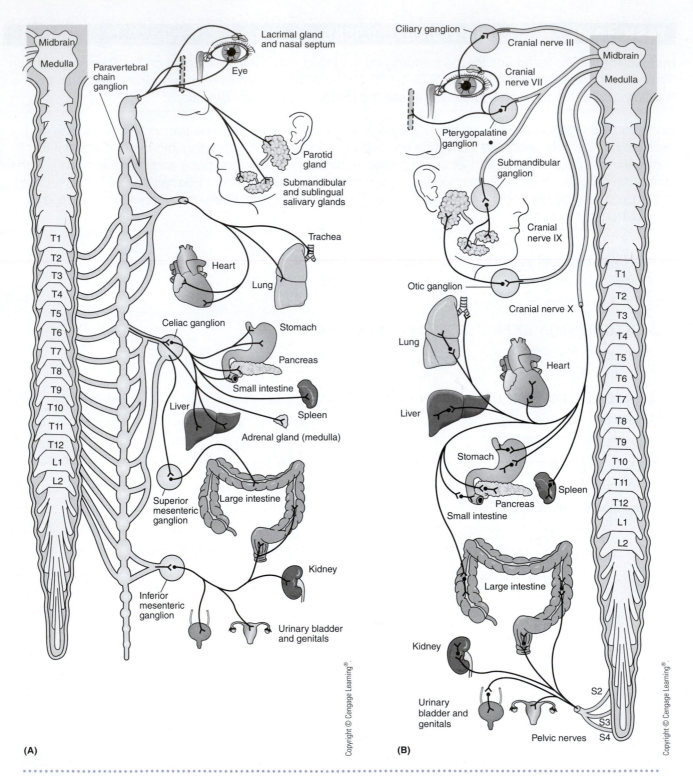

(A)

(B)

FIGURE 10-4 The Nerve Pathways of the Autonomic Nervous System. (A) The Sympathetic Division and (B) the Parasympathetic Division

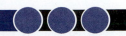

TASK 10-5: SPEECH RECOGNITION EXERCISES

Instructions: The audio files for the following speech recognition exercises are located on the Premium website that accompanies this text (ISBN-13: 978-1-285-73537-5) at http://www.CengageBrain.com. If this is the first time you are registering your account, see the Preface for further instructions.

Once you are logged in to your account, locate the dictation file and Word document for the following speech recognition exercises. Open the audio file to be reviewed according to the exercise number indicated, along with its corresponding Word document. Listen to the dictation and read along with the text, making corrections to the text with regard to formatting, terminology, grammar, spelling, and punctuation. When finished, proofread your work and save the document according to your instructor's directions.

SRT EXERCISE 1: Clinic Note_Report 9013
Patient Name: Jodie Knight
Medical Record Number: 34162

SRT EXERCISE 2: X-Ray Report_Report 3133
Patient Name: Jason Nelson
Medical Record Number: 80032

COMPUTER SOFTWARE **TIPS**

1. At the very bottom of the Word document screen is the status bar, which tells you the page that is currently displayed. You can right-click on the status bar to view a list of options that you can select or deselect to determine which elements appear on the status bar.

2. In Word 2007, Quick Parts and Building Blocks replaced the majority of Autotext. Word 2007 introduced a substitute tool to Autotext. To save text as a Quick Part in Word 2007, highlight the word, sentence, or paragraph, go to the **Insert** toolbar, click **Quick Parts** and select **Save Selection to Quick Parts Gallery** (previously used Quick Parts will appear in the gallery view). A box will appear. Type in the name you wish to use for your automated text, set the Quick Part as **Autotext,** and then press **Save**. The next time you wish to use this text all you need to do is type in the abbreviated name and press F3.

3. The Quick Access Toolbar sits along the top of the Ribbons. This toolbar enables you to set up frequently used icons and actions without having to continuously click through the toolbars.

4. Word has an AutoCorrect option that will automatically capitalize the first letters of sentences for you. To turn it on, press the Microsoft Office button and choose **Word Options** at the bottom of that box. Choose **Proofing** from the list, then **AutoCorrect Options**, and check the appropriate checkbox. Now Word will begin all of your sentences with a capital letter so that you never have to press the shift key again.

5. To quickly see a list of synonyms for a word, highlight a word and right-click (or control-click), select **Synonyms** from the drop-down list, and Word will provide you with a handy list of synonyms for that word. Choose your desired synonym from the list, and Word will automatically insert it in place of the old word.

NEUROLOGY BOOK OF STYLE **TIPS**

1. Typical terms found in an electroencephalogram (EEG) report include: alpha, beta, delta, or theta waves; slow or fast activity; photic stimulation; epileptiform discharges; Hz; K complexes; lateralizing focus; sharp waves; sleep spindles; spike-and-wave pattern; attenuation; symmetric sleep spindles; and amplitude.

2. Cranial nerves can be written in arabic or roman numerals, though you should follow your employer's preference. However, cranial nerves written with ordinals should always use arabic numerals.

    Cranial nerves II-XII are intact.

    Cranial nerves 2-12 are intact.

    The patient has a deficit of the 10th cranial nerve.

3. When transcribing vertebral terminology, use a hyphen to express the space between two vertebrae. It is not necessary to repeat the same letter before the second vertebra, unless preferred by the dictator.

    L1-2 or L1-L2

    C7-T1

However, you should repeat the letter before each numbered vertebra in a list.

The patient had surgery involving L1, L2, L3, and L4.

not

The patient had surgery involving L1, 2, 3, and 4.

4. Nerve conduction studies (including motor and sensory nerve conduction) use measures that include milliseconds (ms), millivolts (mV), and microvolts (mcV).

5. The Glasgow coma scale is the scoring system used most widely to quantify a patient's level of consciousness following a brain injury. It is used routinely by medical personnel to objectively describe a patient's neurologic status. The word "Glasgow" is written in initial caps, and the words "coma" and "scale" (or "score") are written in lowercase. Each parameter of the score is written in arabic numbers.

    The patient had a Glasgow coma score of 8 on admission, which eventually rose to a score of 15 by the time of discharge.

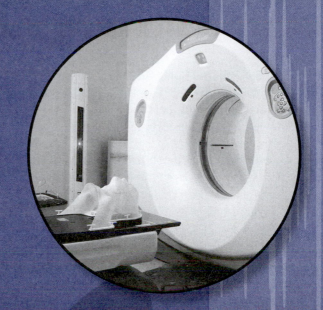

PROJECT 11

Oncology

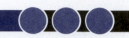

TASK 11-1A: MEDICAL COMPREHENSION EXERCISE

Instructions: Read the clinic note below and answer the questions that follow by choosing the correct letter answer.

FOLLOWUP CLINIC VISIT

PATIENT IDENTIFICATION: Mr. Wolf is a 45-year-old gentleman with a small-cell carcinoma of the larynx. The patient has completed chemotherapy of cisplatin and VP-16 followed by radiation to the larynx. He then received 2 additional cycles of treatment and presents to clinic today for routine followup. Today is day #7 of his treatment.

INTERVAL HISTORY: The patient reports, in general, he feels his throat is healing. However, he did forget to take the Emend with the last cycle of therapy and had a pretty rough weekend, with poor appetite and energy. Patient reports that he has continued to have difficulties taking in adequate p.o. He relates this to poor taste and burning. He says he is drinking a milkshake that is really more of an icy-type drink. He was able to eat an omelet with cheese.

REVIEW OF SYSTEMS: Patient, again, has primary difficulty with oral intake. He feels that perhaps his throat is healing a bit but still is not terribly interested in food. He states he has altered taste. The patient also reports a lower energy over the past week. The patient is not at all concerned about the weight loss, which has been another 7 pounds this past week. This is in excess of more than 50 pounds in weight loss. Today he attempted to tell me that he was wearing lighter clothes, that he had lost a lot of fluid weight, and he did not feel that this was any real weight loss or a problem at all. He apparently is quite happy to take off the weight. The patient's sister and mother, however, feel that he is quite gaunt appearing.

PHYSICAL EXAMINATION: Temperature is 36.3, pulse 82, respirations 18, blood pressure 130/82, weight 82.7 kg, which represents a 3.5 kg weight loss in the past week. In general, he is well appearing though quite thin. He does not appear toxic. He appears comfortable and in no distress. HEENT: He has total alopecia. TMs show normal landmarks without erythema. Sclerae clear. PERRLA. EOMs intact. Funduscopic exam shows normal vasculature. Oral cavity shows some continued erythema of the uvula. The posterior pharynx is remarkably improved. The patient has no evidence of thrush at this time. There are no ulcerations noted. Neck without palpable adenopathy. He does still have the persistent right anterior goiter. Chest shows symmetrical respiratory movements. Lungs are clear to auscultation. Cardiac exam shows regular rate and rhythm without murmurs, rubs, or gallops. Abdomen is soft and nontender. There is no HSM or masses noted. There is no suprapubic or CVA tenderness. Spine is nontender to palpation. Extremities are without edema. Calves are nontender. Neurologic exam is grossly intact.

DIAGNOSTIC STUDIES: WBC 6980, ANC 5730, hemoglobin 12.9, hematocrit 39.6, and platelets 219,000.

ASSESSMENT AND PLAN: The patient is day 7 status post his second cycle of cisplatin and VP-16. We did discuss again extensively the need for increasing caloric intake. I offered suggestions for different types of food groups and that he really needed to be monitoring total caloric intake. Patient adamantly refuses to use any protein supplements but states that he will attempt to increase his protein intake through regular food groups. At the patient's request, we have ordered a cholesterol panel during his next visit. He apparently has previously been on Lipitor. Baseline blood work will also be obtained at that time.

1. A gaunt appearance can be a symptom of _____
   A. macular degeneration.
   B. obesity.
   C. malnourishment.
   D. thrombocytopenia.

2. The posterior pharynx is located at the _____ of the throat.
   A. front
   B. back
   C. bottom
   D. side

3. How does the physician know the patient has no adenopathy?
   A. He cannot feel it.
   B. He cannot see it.
   C. He is assuming the patient does not have it.
   D. Any of the above are correct.

4. What is the purpose of administering cisplatin, VP-16, and radiation to the patient?
   A. To increase the patient's nutrition
   B. To lower the patient's cholesterol levels
   C. To kill the cancer cells
   D. To increase the patient's white cell count

5. The term *alopecia* means _____
   A. that the patient has no color in his face.
   B. that the patient is bald.
   C. that the patient is blind.
   D. that the patient's skin has an erythematous hue.

6. Where is the patient's goiter located?
   A. In the back on the right side
   B. In the front on the left side
   C. In the back on the left side
   D. In the front on the right side

7. In this report, what does "ANC" stand for?
   A. Absolute neutrophil count
   B. Acid neutralizing capacity
   C. Antineutrophil cytoplasm
   D. Ancillary

8. "EOMs" refer to the _____
   A. sclerae.
   B. pupil.
   C. rods and cones of the retina.
   D. muscles of the eye.

9. What is one of the doctor's concerns about the patient?
   A. His neurologic status
   B. His baldness
   C. His lack of caloric intake
   D. His high blood pressure

10. Why is the patient taking Lipitor?
    A. He has high blood pressure.
    B. He has high cholesterol.
    C. He has elevated liver function studies.
    D. He has a poor iron binding capacity.

11. What does "HSM" refer to?
    A. The liver and spleen
    B. The spleen only
    C. The kidneys
    D. The pancreas

12. Why is the patient taking Emend?
    A. For his low caloric intake
    B. For his low hemoglobin
    C. For nausea and vomiting
    D. For elevated white counts

13. Where is this cancer located?
    A. In the throat
    B. In the neck
    C. In the cervical spine
    D. In the back of the head

14. How many days has it been since the patient's last chemotherapy?
    A. 10
    B. 1
    C. 7
    D. 16

15. What did the physician observe about the uvula?
    A. It is persistently swollen.
    B. It is persistently red.
    C. It is persistently pale.
    D. It is again normal in appearance.

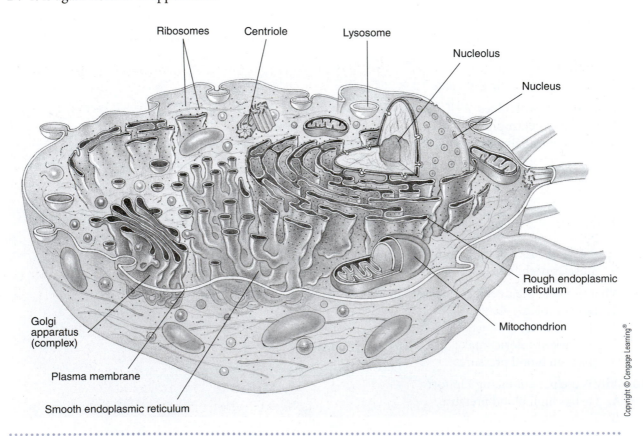

FIGURE 11-1 The Cell

TASK 11-1B: COMBINING FORMS EXERCISE

Instructions: Next to each combining form, write its meaning.

1. carcin/o _____

2. heredit/o _____

3. cyt/o _____

4. nucle/o _____

5. cellul/o _____

6. mit/o _____

7. lys/o _____

8. invas/o _____

9. chrom/o _____

10. mutat/o _____

TASK 11-1C: MATCHING EXERCISE

Instructions: Match the cancer in the first column with its definition in the right column.

1. _____ astrocytoma	A. A cancer found in the top layer of the skin.
2. _____ meningioma	B. A disease in which cancerous cells are found in the tissues under the skin or mucous membranes that line the mouth, nose and anus; often found in patients with AIDS.
3. _____ acoustic neuroma	C. Cancer of the branching cell that supports neurons in the cerebrum of the brain.
4. _____ ductal carcinoma	D. A malignant tumor found in bone or soft tissue, mainly affecting adolescents.
5. _____ Ewing sarcoma	E. A cancer of the blood or bone marrow.
6. _____ melanoma	F. Cancer of melanocytes of the skin.
7. _____ basal cell carcinoma	G. A noncancerous tumor that develops on the nerve that connects the ear to the brain.
8. _____ medulloblastoma	H. A type of cancer that starts in bones.
9. _____ fibroma	I. A tumor of the cerebellum formed from poorly developed cells; sometimes referred to as a "PNET."
10. _____ osteosarcoma	J. Cancer of a blood vessel or lymphatic vessel.
11. _____ Kaposi sarcoma	K. A tumor arising from the membranous layers surrounding the central nervous system.
12. _____ multiple myeloma	L. A type of tumor that presents in the duct of a gland.
13. _____ Hodgkin lymphoma	M. A type of cancer that is formed by malignant plasma cells.
14. _____ leukemia	N. A cancer of the lymph system that results from abnormal lymphocytes called Reed-Sternberg cells.
15. _____ angiosarcoma	O. A tumor made up of fibrous connective tissue as opposed to cancerous cells.

TASK 11-2: PROOFREADING EXERCISES

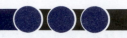

Instructions: The proofreading documents below are designed to challenge your proofreading and editing skills. The documents may contain missing demographic information, incorrect headings, misspelled words, misplaced punctuation, and other errors within the document. Read each report below and identify the error by circling the word. Then retype the document with the corrected text and formatting. When finished, proofread your work and save the document to your student disk using a different file name.

PROOFREADING EXERCISE 1

FOLLOWUP CLINIC VISIT

PATIENT IDENTIFICATION: The patient is a 65-year-old woman with metastic invasive ducal carcinoma of the breast, metastatic to her bones.

INTERVAL HISTORY: The patient has been doing relatively well since her last appointment with me. She has intermittent bony pain secondary to her bone metastasis but has been continuing to take her arimidex and Zometa as prescribed. She complains of right femor pain and left-sided rib pain, both in the areas of known metastasis. This, she states, has improved somewhat since originally being diagnosed and has not worsened in intensity. She denies any fevers no shortness of breath, no cough, no constipation, no diarrhea. She denies any dysuria. She does have some frequency in urination at night, possibly secondary to her hydroclorthiazide.

MEDICATIONS: Arimidex 1 mg daily, oxycodone 5 mg every six hours as needed for pain, Flonase 50 mcg as needed, Atarax 25 mg daily, Lipitor 20 mcg daily, and hydrochlorothiazide 125 mg daily.

REVIEW OF SYSTEMS: As above.

PHYSICAL EXAMINATION: She is a well-appearing woman in no apparent distress. She is afebrile at 369, heart rate 81, blood pressure 109/75, respiratory rate 18, body surface area 1.6. Pupils equal, round, and reactive to light and accommodation. Extraocular movements are intact. She has no cervical lymphadenopathy. Oral pharynx is clear. Chest was clear to auscultation. She has some moderate kyfosis. Heart is regular rate and rhythm. There is no superclavicular adenopathy noted. She has some tenderness over the left rib sights, most notably over T8-9. No CTA tenderness. Her abdominal tenderness is soft, nontender, and nondistended. No hepatosplenomegaly was noted. She has chronic lymphedema of the lower extremities, left slightly greater than right, which is unchanged from her prior physical exam.

DIAGNOSTIC STUDIES: Her laboratory results today show calcium of 10.3, BUN 13, creatinine 0.9, and her LFT's are within normal limits. Her hemoglobin is 13.6 with a white count of 8.30 and platelet count of 237,000.

(Continues)

PROOFREADING EXERCISE 1 *(Continued)*

CT scans to reevaluate her disease revealed some interval appearance of medial stinal fibrosis compatible with her radiation therapy. She has interval decrease in her left internal mamary lymph node since her prior exam. She has stable tiny nodularity of the left lung apex and a stable CT scan of her abdomen.

ASSESSMENT/AND PLAN: The patient, her daughter, and I spoke at length regarding preceeding forward with her care. We will continue her Arimidex 1 mg daily as she seems to have had good response to this with some decrease in the size of her lymphadenopathy and shown some minimal improvement in her bony pain. We will also continue with the Zometa 4 mg iv monthly and I will follow up with her in 3 months time to reevaluate her with CT scans.

PROOFREADING EXERCISE 2

CLINIC VISIT

PATIENT IDENTIFICATION: Mr. Mitchell is 76-year-old gentleman with metastatic recurrent rectal cancer on FOLFOX, Avastin, and Tarceva, who is being seen for follow up today. He is to start cycle 2 day 15 tomorrow.

INTREVAL HISTORY: Since he was last seen, he has been doing fairly well. He had an episode of some dizziness while getting the Avastin and when we have done EKG's periodically, he has been in Wenkeback rhythm where he will have a skipped beat every forth atrial contraction or so. I do not think this is a dangerous rhythm by any means but I did ask him to stop his lopressor and we are following him fairly closely with regular EKGs. He has had no symptoms, but he seems to get episodes of dizziness after the Avastin and so for this reason, we are going to hold the next Avastin doze.

He continues to have a suprapubic catheter and I examined it today, and it looks as thought he is having a lot of skin breakdown in the area. I am pretty concerned about it and clearly, the dressing had not been changed and the guaze was foul smelling and very dark. He says he has a hard time seeing the area and thus I have paged the study nurse to see if we can set up home nursing to come out and help him change the dressing and help follow this. He does have a stricture in his urethera and he will be having that addressed surgically by the urology service. His colstomy is working well in his right lower quadrant and his superpubic tube appears to be working well from a functional standpoint.

MEDICATIONS:

1. Colace 100 mg by mouth 2 times per day.
2. Actos 30 mg by mouth daily.
3. Allopurinol 300 mg by mouth daily. I am going to check to see there is no interaction with 5/FU.
4. Diovan 80,12.5 mg by mouth daily.

(Continues)

PROOFREADING EXERCISE 2 *(Continued)*

5. Aspirin 325 mcg daily.
6. Oxycodone 5 mg every 4-6 hours as needed.
7. Doxizosin 400 mg by mouth daily.

PHYSICAL EXAMINATION: The patient is in no parent distress. He looks well. Temperature 36.8, blood pressure 88 over 66 but he is not having any dizziness, heart rate 90, respiratory rate 18, weight 119.7 kg, which compares to previous weight of 121 mg. HEENT: Normocephalic and atraumatic. Pupils equal, round, and reactive to light. Extraoccular movements are intact. Oropharynx is clear. Neck is supple without lymphadenopathy, JVD, or thyrmegaly. Chest is clear to auscultation bilaterally. Cardiovascular exam is regular rate and rhythm, normal s1 and s2. no murmurs, rubs, or gallops. Abdomen exam shows normal bowel sounds, nontender, nondistended, no hepasplenomegaly. His colostomy in his left lower quadrant is functioning well. His suprapubic tube, which is just right of the midline, has a foul smelling dressing that is not properly changed. I personally changed the dressing and put a fresh 1 on today. There is about a 1.5 cm area of skin breakdown around the tube but it does not appear to be actively infection. We will be arranging for some home care to take care of that dressing. Extremities showed no clubbing or cyanotic. He does have trace symmetric edema. Skin exam shows no rash. Neurologic exam shows he is alert and orientated times 3. He is pleasant. Cranial nerves 2-12 are grossly intact. He ambulates without difficulty.

DIAGNOSTIC STUDIES: A comprehensive chemistry panel is normal except for an albumin which is slightly low at 3.3. His troponin and MB is negative. His white count is 4500, hematocrit 20, platelet count 259, INR 1.10.

ASSESSMENT AND PLAN: In summary, this is a 76-year-old gentleman with recurrent metastatic rectal cancer with liver metastases who is on protocol J0220, which is FOLFOX combined with Tarceva and Avastin. He has tolerated chemotherapy fairly well. Although he has had dizziness after getting the Avastin; and for this reason, we will hold it with the next dose. After this next course of treatment, he will finish two cycles and we will get a scan and go from there. We are all eager to have his urethral stricture taken care of so we can get his suprapubic tubes out, so we may need to hold his chemotherapy a bit after cycle 2 so that he can have this done. I am especially concerned about the skin breakdown over the suprapubic tube. I think we need to be aggressive about getting rid of it. He will follow up in 30 day.

ONCOLOGY TRANSCRIPTION **TIPS**

1. "Radio" words are one word: *radiosurgery*, *radionuclide*, *radiograph* (another name for x-ray).

2. The word *woody* is often used in dictation to describe skin texture that is hard, rough, and thickened after receiving surgical or radiation treatment.

3. The term *patent* means "open." Physicians use this word a lot to describe clear vessels, arteries, and unobstructed openings (the noun form of the word is *patency*). Do not transcribe this as "patient" or "parent".

4. Do not assume the short-form word "heme" means Hemoccult. Hemoccult is the brand name of a fecal occult blood test kit used by physicians. This term is capitalized when used in dictation. *Heme* is a compound of blood but is used sometimes in place of the word "blood."

> The patient's *Hemoccult* test was negative.
>
> *but*
>
> The patient had *heme-positive stools*.
> (*not* Hemoccult positive)

5. You may hear a physician use a term that sounds like "b-c-r, able." This refers to a genetic abnormality common to leukemia patients. These patients have what is called the Philadelphia chromosome, a defective chromosome called *Abl* involving a gene called *Bcr*. These terms combine to form the *bcr/ablgene*, which, when dictated, is transcribed in all lowercase letters.

TASK 11-3: CLOZE EXERCISES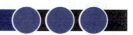

Instructions: The audio files for the following cloze exercises are located on the Premium website that accompanies this text (ISBN-13: 978-1-285-73537-5) at http://www.CengageBrain.com. If this is the first time you are registering your account, see the Preface for further instructions.

Once you are logged in to your account, locate the dictation file and Word document for the following cloze exercises. Open the audio file to be reviewed according to the exercise number indicated, along with its corresponding Word document. Listen to the dictation and read along with the text, filling in the missing words in the report by thinking critically and analytically about the context of the text you are reading. When finished, proofread your work and save the document according to your instructor's directions.

CLOZE EXERCISE 1: Discharge Summary_Report 7
Patient Name: Lien Change
Medical Record Number: 15128

CLOZE EXERCISE 2: Chest X-ray and Isotope Bone Scan_Report 11
Patient Name: Virginia Haynes
Medical Record Number: 38135

TASK 11-4: TRANSCRIPTION EXERCISES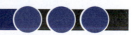

Instructions: The audio files for the following transcription exercises are located on the Premium website that accompanies this text (ISBN-13: 978-1-285-73537-5) at http://www.CengageBrain.com. If this is the first time you are registering your account, see the Preface for further instructions.

Once you are logged in to your account, locate and open the audio file to be transcribed according to the exercise number indicated and transcribe each report. Do not insert a heading into the document if the text requires a second page, but let the text wrap naturally to the second page and continue typing. Transcribe the reports using the formatting specifics indicated in the Document Formatting Guidelines located at the beginning of this book. When finished, proofread your work and save the document according to your instructor's directions.

TRANSCRIPTION EXERCISE 1: Discharge Summary_Report 4

Patient Name: Ty Simmons
Medical Record Number: 10642

TRANSCRIPTION EXERCISE 2: Operative Note_Report 9

Patient Name: Jacob Smith
Medical Record Number: 98009

TRANSCRIPTION EXERCISE 3: Letter_Report 15

Patient Name: Margaret Jenkins
Medical Record Number: 33905

TRANSCRIPTION EXERCISE 4: Discharge Summary_Report 7

Patient Name: Sarah Jennings
Medical Record Number: 28218

TRANSCRIPTION EXERCISE 5: Abdominal Sonogram_Report 3385

Patient Name: Vernon Griffin
Medical Record Number: 71573

TASK 11-5: SPEECH RECOGNITION EXERCISES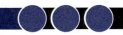

Instructions: The audio files for the following speech recognition exercises are located on the Premium website that accompanies this text (ISBN-13: 978-1-285-73537-5) at http://www.CengageBrain.com. If this is the first time you are registering your account, see the Preface for further instructions.

Once you are logged in to your account, locate the dictation file and Word document for the following speech recognition exercises. Open the audio file to be reviewed according to the exercise number indicated, along with its corresponding Word document. Listen to the dictation and read along with the text, making corrections to the text with regard to formatting, terminology, grammar, spelling, and punctuation. When finished, proofread your work and save the document according to your instructor's directions.

SRT EXERCISE 1: Clinic Note_Report 6

Patient Name: Lee Wong
Medical Record Number: 40506

SRT EXERCISE 2: Clinic Note_Report 9039

Patient Name: Andrew Hughes
Medical Record Number: 60998

SRT EXERCISE 3: Clinic Note_Report 6196
Patient Name: Samuel Erinne
Medical Record Number: 37756

SRT EXERCISE 4: Clinic Note_Report 9045
Patient Name: Sandra McKeown
Medical Record Number: 16110

COMPUTER SOFTWARE **TIPS**

1. If you copy and paste a lot of content from different sources—other Word documents or Outlook e-mail messages, the formatting of the original document text may be carried over to your document. To avoid this, highlight and copy (or cut). Then on the **Home** ribbon, click the **Paste** button. Choose **Paste Special** and **Unformatted Text** in the list of choices. This will save time in having to reformat the pasted text.

2. Word 2007 will add a space between paragraphs by default. To turn off the space between paragraphs, on the **Home** ribbon, find the **Paragraph** section. In the bottom right corner of that section, click on the arrow to open the **Paragraph** dialog box. In the dialog box, choose the box that says "Don't add space between paragraphs of the same style." Click OK.

3. You can quickly change text that has similar formatting. First position your cursor in a section of the document containing the formatting characteristics you are looking for (for example, 14-point Times New Roman text). On the **Home** ribbon, access the **Editing** section, click **Select,** and then choose **Select Text with Similar Formatting**. Once you have selected the text bearing the formatting, you can change it using the options on the **Home** ribbon. Word will change the formatting of all similar text in all locations throughout the document.

4. Word contains dozens of shortcut keys, and it is difficult to remember them all. To display the shortcut keys in Word, display them in Screen Tips. First click the **Microsoft Office** button and choose **Word Options** at the bottom of the box. Open the **Advance** tab. In the **Display** section, select **Show shortcut keys in Screen Tips** and click OK. Now when you hold the mouse pointer over a command button on one of the ribbons, a box will appear showing the command and the shortcut key for that command.

5. To keep a table row from breaking between pages, do the following: First select the row you want to keep together on the same page. Locate the **Layout** ribbon and select the **Table Tools** tab. Click **Properties** to open the **Table Properties** dialog box. Check the Row tab, then deselect the check box that says **Allow row to break across page**. Then click OK. Now rows will stay on the same page and not break between pages.

ONCOLOGY BOOK OF STYLE **TIPS**

1. Cancer is quantified by staging and grading. Cancer stage is written with the word "stage" in lowercase letters followed by a roman numeral, from 0 to IV. Subdivisions of the stage are written by adding capital letters followed by arabic numbers, much like an outline tree, without spaces or hyphens.

   The patient has stage II adenocarcinoma of the cecum.

   The patient's cancer has progressed to stage IIIA2.

   Express the grade of the cancer with the word "grade" written in lowercase followed by arabic numerals from 1 to 4.

   The patient was diagnosed with stage I, grade 2 carcinoma of the left breast.

2. Cancers expressed by using the TNM staging system for malignant tumor staging is transcribed with no spaces between the letter and the number, and no space between each letter designation. An uppercase "X" next to the letter indicates that a parameter could not be assessed.

   The patient has T1N0MX cancer of the larynx.

   See the *Book of Style, 3rd Ed.*, for a further discussion of the TNM system and its subcategories.

3. The Dukes system is used to classify cancers relating to the colon or rectum. It is transcribed using the word *Dukes* followed by a capital letter, and subdivided by arabic numbers with no spaces in between. Do not use an apostrophe with the word *Dukes*. The term is *Dukes*, not "Duke's" or "Duke."

   Dukes A carcinoma

   Dukes C3 cancer

4. Physicians often will revert to acronyms when dictating about cancer trials as well as treatments. For example, physicians may pronounce the S-W-O-G trial as "swog" and the E-C-O-G trial as "E-cog". Treatments may sound like "CHOP" (**c**yclophosphamide, **h**ydroxydaunorubicin, **O**ncovin, and **p**rednisone) or "MOPP" (**m**ethotrexate, **v**incristine, **p**rednisone and **p**rocarbazine).

5. *Centigray* is a unit of absorbed radiation by body tissues and should be transcribed in its abbreviated form, cGy (if dictated as "centigray") or Gy (if dictated as "gray").

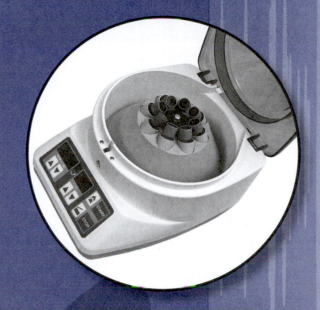

PROJECT 12

Immunology

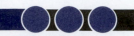

TASK 12-1A: MATCHING EXERCISE

Instructions: Match the following immunologic disorders in the left column with their corresponding definitions in the right column. Each definition should be used only once.

Term	Definition
1. _____ lymphoma	A. An overactivity of the thyroid gland.
2. _____ Graves disease	B. A chronic autoimmune disorder that causes skin to harden and scar.
3. _____ psoriasis	C. A multisystem autoimmune disease characterized by achy joints; inflammation of the fibrous tissue surrounding the heart; unexplained rashes on the face, neck, or scalp; and other disorders.
4. _____ HIV-G	D. A form of vasculitis that affects primarily the lungs, kidneys, and upper respiratory tract.
5. _____ rheumatoid arthritis	E. A chronic autoimmune disease in which a person's white blood cells attack their moisture-producing glands, causing dry eyes, dry mouth, and other symptoms.
6. _____ vasculitis	F. An inflammatory disease of the nervous system that disrupts communication between the brain and other parts of the body by forming plaques on portions of the sheaths surrounding the neurons of the brain and spinal cord.
7. _____ Hashimoto thyroiditis	
8. _____ Sjögren syndrome	
9. _____ Wegener granulomatosis	G. The virus that infects and destroys T cells, paving the way for other infections and cancers to enter the body.
10. _____ scleroderma	H. A condition that involves inflammation in the blood vessels due to the immune system attacking those vessels by mistake.
11. _____ systemic lupus erythematosus	I. Causes chronic inflammation of blood vessels throughout the body.
12. _____ multiple sclerosis	J. Blood vessels in the fingers become narrow, diminishing blood supply and causing fingers to become pale, waxy-white, or purple in cold temperatures.
13. _____ Raynaud phenomenon	K. A condition that occurs when antibodies attack the thyroid gland directly, leading to insufficient production of thyroid hormone.
14. _____ polyarthritis	L. An autoimmune disorder in which the immune system attacks and causes inflammation of the joints and surrounding tissues of the body.
15. _____ Behçet disease	M. An autoimmune condition featuring thickening of the skin with associated redness and scaling.
	N. A general term for a group of cancers that originate in the lymphocytes.
	O. Inflammation and soft tissue swelling of many joints at the same time.

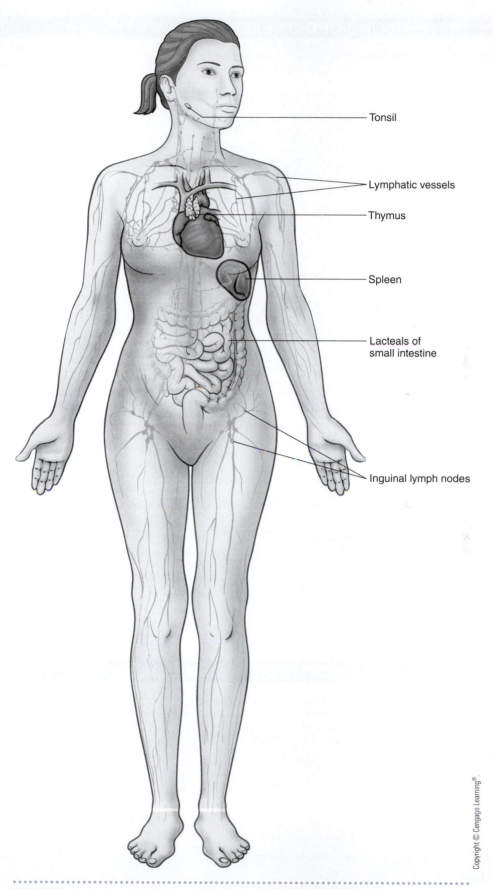

- Tonsil
- Lymphatic vessels
- Thymus
- Spleen
- Lacteals of small intestine
- Inguinal lymph nodes

FIGURE 12-1 The Vessels and Organs of the Lymphatic System

TASK 12-1B: SPELLING CHOICE EXERCISE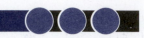

Instructions: Choose the correct spelling of each immunologic term.

1.	erythematosis	erythematosus	erythemetosus
2.	lymfocite	lymphcite	lymphocyte
3.	thimus	thymus	thymis
4.	reumatoid	rhumatoid	rheumatoid
5.	vermiform	vermaform	virmaform
6.	lupus	leupus	lupis
7.	hemolitic	hemolytic	hemalytic
8.	antagen	antigen	antigin
9.	antebody	antibodey	antibody
10.	immunoglobulin	imunoglobbulin	immunoglobulen
11.	autoimune	autoimmune	autoimunne
12.	pathigen	pathogin	pathogen
13.	skleroderma	scleroderma	scleraderma
14.	apheresis	aferesis	aphiresis
15.	antecardiolipn	anticardiolipin	anticardilipin
16.	nutropenia	neutropinia	neutropenia
17.	compliment	complimment	complement
18.	reseptors	receptors	recepters
19.	sclerodactyly	scleradactily	sclerodactoly
20.	granulomatosis	grannulomatosus	granulomotosis

TASK 12-1C: MEDICAL WORD BUILDING EXERCISE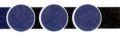

Instructions: Complete the following sentences by creating the correct term using the following word parts.

aden/o	-pathy
immun/o	-logy
leuk/o	-ectomy
lymph/o	-itis
myel/o	-oma
cyt/o	-osis
tonsill/o	-emia
lymphaden/o	
splen/o	

1. The study of immune system is called _____.

2. The surgical removal of the tonsils is called _____.

3. The study of cell structure is called _____.

4. A type of cancer arising from plasma cells is called _____.

5. A cancer of the blood is called _____.

6. The inflammation of the clumps of tissue located at the back of the nasal passages is called _____.

7. A general term for cancers that originate in the lymphocytes is called _____.

8. A condition in which there is more than the usual number of cells is called _____.

9. The enlargement or swelling of the lymph nodes is called _____.

10. The surgical removal of the spleen is called _____.

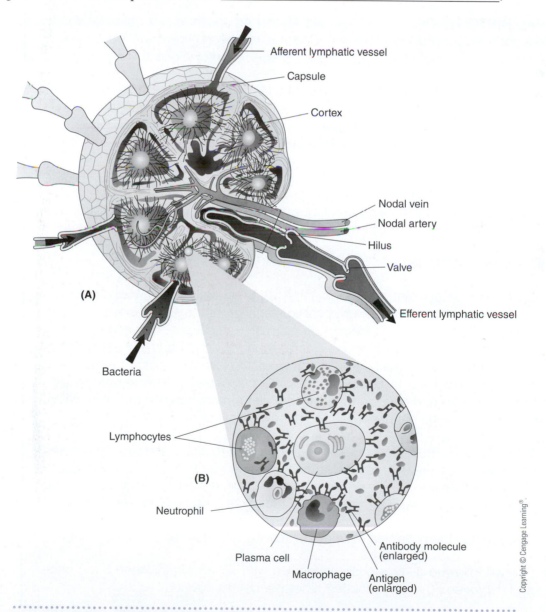

FIGURE 12-2 Lymph Node (A) Cross-section Showing the Flow of Lymph, and (B) Microscopic Detail of Bacteria being Destroyed within the Lymph Node

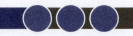

TASK 12-2: PROOFREADING EXERCISES

Instructions: The proofreading documents below are designed to challenge your proofreading and editing skills. The documents may contain missing demographic information, incorrect headings, misspelled words, misplaced punctuation, and other errors within the document. Read each report below and identify the error by circling the word. Then retype the document with the corrected text and formatting. When finished, proofread your work and save the document to your student disk using a different file name.

PROOFREADING EXERCISE 1

CLINIC NOTE

REASON FOR VISIT: SLE.

INTERVAL HISTORY: This is a 29-year-old African American female with sle who is here today for a scheduled follow/up visit. She was last seen here in the lupus clinic a month ago with worsening arthralgias and had received Triamcinolone 100 mg injection.

The patient states that she did feel improvement after the triamcinolone infection. However, she started with increase in pain in both her knees and elbows since the last 2 to 3 days. She does state that her ankle pain has improved. However, she continues to have morning stiffness for about 10 to 15 min in the morning. She denies any ulcers or rashes.

Her SLE was diagnosed five years ago and has been characterized by lympdenopathy, arthralgias, arthritis, pleuritis, paracarditis, lupus anticoagulant and anti-double-stranded DNA, anti-Smith, ANA with a titer of 1,280, low C-4, low C3, and a history of a miscarriage.

CURRENT MEDICATIONS: She is on Plaquenil 400 mcg once per day.

FINDINGS: On physical exam, the weight is 191.3, temperature 98.1, blood pressure 113/73, and pain is 10 over 10. On physical examination of the skin, there is no rash. Head and neck exam reveals no ulcers and no thrush. Lungs demonstrate bilateral air entry. Heart sounds: S1S2 are audible, regular rate and rhythm. Abdominal exam shows she is soft nontender, and bowel sounds are present. On extremity exam, there is trace edema with nontender calfs. A comprehensive musculoskeletal exam reveals tenderness in bilateral elbows and knees and also some warmth are noted in both the wrists. However, there is no signs of arthralgias. Neurologically she is nonfocal.

ASSESSMENT: SLE. The patient does have significant arthralgias and a recently noted low C4 value. She has already received a triamcinolone injection of 100 mg ten days back and she continues to have arthralgias. She will be started on prednisone 5 mg once per day and also she was advised to start naproxen 500 mg 2 times per day with food. She is not a candidate for methatrexate at this time because there are no obvious signs of sinovitis. On the physician estimate of activity, she received a 1 under joints.

PLAN: She will followup as previously scheduled. We will add prednisone 5 mg once per day and naproxen 50 mg by mouth 2 times per day as adviced.

PROOFREADING EXERCISE 2

CLINIC NOTE

REASON FOR VISIT: SLE.

HISTORY OF PRESENT ILLNESS: This 32-year-old Caucasian female comes in for routine followup. She mentions some morning stiffness that is not any worse from previous visits. She also has had 2 episodes of either lower back pain or hip pain in the last 7 months. Most recently was 2 weeks ago and it lasted about 2 weeks, this is slowly resolving. She did actually have bilateral hip MRIs, which was completely negative. Although a large ovarian cyst was seen and she is currently being treated with a Nuva ring for this.

The patient has never had a DEXA scan done. She does mention that she was on prednisone in childhood for about 6 years for Crohn's disease. We mentioned that this would be appropriate to have as a test for her to due, and we have given her an order to get this done at her next visit.

MEDICATIONS: Plaquenil 400, naproxen 500 2 times per day as needed, aspirin 81 mg, Lexapro 10, amitriptyline 10, Tylenol p.m. as needed.

FINDINGS: On physical exam, the weight is 160 pounds, temperature 99.1 degrees f., blood pressure 121/65, pain 0/10. On physical examination of the skin, there is no rash or alopecia present. She does have some acne present and will be follow up with a dermatologist. On HEENT:there is no oral or nasal ulcers and no thrush present. On chest exam, she is clear to auscultation bilaterally. Cardiac exam reveals regular rate and rhythm without murmurs, rubs, or gallops. Abdominal exam shows she is soft, non-tender, nondistended. On extremity exam, there is no clubbing, cyanosis, or edema. On comprehensive musculoskeletal exam, she does have some arthralgias of her MCP's and knees, there is no synovitis present. Neurologically she is nonfocal.

ASSESSMENT:

1. SLA with arthralgias. On the physician estimate of activity, she scores a 1 with a one for joints.
2. She does have some fascial acne. She will follow up with a dermatologist. I do not think that it is related to any of her current medications. Her dermatologist certainly may try her on Metrgel or minicycline.
3. We do recommend a dexa scan as she has never had one done and she was on chronic prednisone use in childhood.
4. She has had these episodes of lower back pain and questionable hip pain. At the next occurence, we asked her to contact the office and we would consider medication such as Flexeril as a muscle relaxant to see if some of this is due to muscle spasm.

PLAN: Follow up in three months.

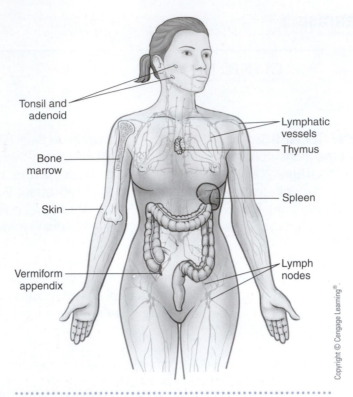

Copyright © Cengage Learning®

FIGURE 12-3 Lymphoid Tissue Structures Play an Important Role in the Immune System

 IMMUNOLOGY TRANSCRIPTION **TIPS**

1. The term *shotty* refers to something hard and round, like shotgun pellets. It is commonly used to describe the feel of lymph nodes when they are palpated, or felt, through the skin resembling shotgun pellets. Do not mistranscribe this term as "shoddy," which means something that is made of inferior material or workmanship.

2. When a physician dictates abbreviations like "I-G-M" or "I-G-A" in a medical document, an antibody is what is being referred, and this abbreviation is transcribed using a combination of capital and small letters, such as *IgM* or *IgA*.

3. Note the immunologic disease *Graves disease* does not contain an apostrophe. The correct transcription is *Graves disease*, not "Grave's disease" or "Graves' disease."

4. Chemotherapy combination treatments used in diseases like lymphoma are sometimes referred to as *regimens* or *protocols* in dictation. Listen carefully and always verify the combination dictated, as it is easy to confuse many regimens used for different diseases. For example, the protocol ABVD is not the same chemical combination as AVDP or EBVP.

5. Drugs that slow the progression of autoimmune disease are called disease modifying antirheumatic drugs, or DMARDs. This abbreviation sounds like "DEE-mardz" when dictated by physicians.

TASK 12-3: CLOZE EXERCISES

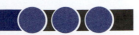

Instructions: The audio files for the following cloze exercises are located on the Premium website that accompanies this text (ISBN-13: 978-1-285-73537-5) at http://www.CengageBrain.com. If this is the first time you are registering your account, see the Preface for further instructions.

Once you are logged in to your account, locate the dictation file and Word document for the following cloze exercises. Open the audio file to be reviewed according to the exercise number indicated, along with its corresponding Word document. Listen to the dictation and read along with the text, filling in the missing words in the report by thinking critically and analytically about the context of the text you are reading. When finished, proofread your work and save the document according to your instructor's directions.

CLOZE EXERCISE 1: Clinic Note_Report 66
Patient Name: Gloria Fields
Medical Record Number: 72230

CLOZE EXERCISE 2: Clinic Note_Report 23
Patient Name: Irene Douglas
Medical Record Number: 64828

TASK 12-4: TRANSCRIPTION EXERCISES

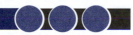

Instructions: The audio files for the following transcription exercises are located on the Premium website that accompanies this text (ISBN-13: 978-1-285-73537-5) at http://www.CengageBrain.com. If this is the first time you are registering your account, see the Preface for further instructions.

Once you are logged in to your account, locate and open the audio file to be transcribed according to the exercise number indicated and transcribe each report. Do not insert a heading into the document if the text requires a second page, but let the text wrap naturally to the second page and continue typing. Transcribe the reports using the formatting specifics indicated in the Document Formatting Guidelines located at the beginning of this book. When finished, proofread your work and save the document according to your instructor's directions.

TRANSCRIPTION EXERCISE 1: Discharge Summary_Report 8
Patient Name: Juanita Jimenez
Medical Record Number: 31110

TRANSCRIPTION EXERCISE 2: Operative Note_Report 6
Patient Name: John Jones
Medical Record Number: 99011

TRANSCRIPTION EXERCISE 3: Clinic Note_Report 10
Patient Name: Heather Dean
Medical Record Number: 66743

TRANSCRIPTION EXERCISE 4: Clinic Note_Report 22
Patient Name: Evelyn Walsh
Medical Record Number: 20112

TRANSCRIPTION EXERCISE 5: Thyroid Sonogram_Report 3363
Patient Name: Martin Cox
Medical Record Number: 11375

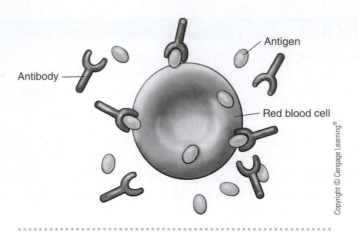

FIGURE 12-4 Antibodies Bind Together Foreign Antigens to Neutralize them and to Flag them for Destruction by the Immune System

TASK 12-5: SPEECH RECOGNITION EXERCISES

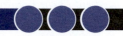

Instructions: The audio files for the following speech recognition exercises are located on the Premium website that accompanies this text (ISBN-13: 978-1-285-73537-5) at http://www.CengageBrain.com. If this is the first time you are registering your account, see the Preface for further instructions.

Once you are logged in to your account, locate the dictation file and Word document for the following speech recognition exercises. Open the audio file to be reviewed according to the exercise number indicated, along with its corresponding Word document. Listen to the dictation and read along with the text, making corrections to the text with regard to formatting, terminology, grammar, spelling, and punctuation. When finished, proofread your work and save the document according to your instructor's directions.

SRT EXERCISE 1: Clinic Note_Report 1
Patient Name: Dante Kennedy
Medical Record Number: 20415

SRT EXERCISE 2: Clinic Note_Report 30
Patient Name: Rachel Beck
Medical Record Number: 22273

COMPUTER SOFTWARE **TIPS**

1. If you do not want automatic numbering to occur with itemized lists, choose the **Microsoft Office** button, then **Word Options** at the bottom of the box. Select **Proofing** view from the left-sided list that appears. Click the **AutoCorrect Options** button, then **AutoFormat As You Type** tab and uncheck the box that says Automatic Bulleted Lists and Automatic Numbered Lists.

2. When working with **columns**, you can quickly review how the columns appear when printed by choosing the **Microsoft Office** button, then **Print Preview**. When finished, click the **Close Print Preview** button on the **Print Preview** tab to return to your document screen.

3. You can create a header or footer quickly by double-clicking over the header and footer areas of the document.

4. To view the top and bottom margins of a document in the Print Layout view, double-click the lines that mark the top and bottom page boundaries. You can also change this setting permanently by choosing the **Microsoft Office** button and choosing **Word Options**. In the **Display** menu on the left, check the box next to **Show White Space Between Pages** to see the space, or unchecking the box to not view the top and bottom margins in the document.

5. The status bar in the lower left corner of the document window shows the number of words in a document as you type. If you want to only see the number of words in a selection of text rather than the entire document, simply select the text and the status bar will indicate how many words your selected text contains out of the entire document word count.

IMMUNOLOGY BOOK OF STYLE **TIPS**

1. *T lymphocytes* (or T cells) and *B lymphocytes* (or B cells) are the most common of leukocytes that carry out antigen-specific immune responses in the body. They should be transcribed in their abbreviated forms and not extended, with no hyphen except when used as an adjective preceding a noun.

   T cells

   B cells

   B-cell count

2. Interferons are proteins made and released by host cells in response to the presence of pathogens in order to fight infection. Generally the word "interferon" is transcribed in lowercase letters with its accompanying Greek letter spelled out. In addition, be aware that "alfa" is the correct spelling of the first Greek letter of the alphabet in this format, not "alpha."

   interferon alfa

   interferon beta

3. Immunoglobulin prefixes are expanded when they are first mentioned in a medical document but abbreviated thereafter.

monomeric IgM	mIgM
membrane-bound IgM	mIgM
surface IgM	sIgM
surface IgA	sIgA

4. Every cell in the body carries distinctive marker molecules called *human leukocyte antigen* (HLA) that determine tissue type, which is used for transplant purposes. These markers are expressed with a combination of upper and lowercase letters and hyphens.

   HLA-B27

   HLA-DR5

   HLA-DRw10

5. *Clusters of differentiation*, or CDs, refer to the classification system for identifying cellular surface antigens. These terms should be transcribed by typing CD in all capital letters, along with lowercase subclassification letters and symbols.

   CD10

   CD4

   CD20

APPENDIX A

HELPFUL MEDICAL TRANSCRIPTION WEBSITES

Name	Site	Description
AHDI	http://www.ahdionline.org	The professional organization that sets the standards for education and practice in the field of medical transcription.
Google	http://www.google.com/cse/home?cx=010964806533120826279%3Akyuedntb2fy&hl=en	A Google MT Word Seeker search engine that searches only health and medical transcription websites as well as employment opportunities.
LabCorp	https://www.labcorp.com/wps/portal/provider/testmenu/	A listing of lab tests associated with different diseases.
Medical Lexicon	http://www.medilexicon.com/medicalabbreviations.php	A database of medical abbreviations and acronyms.
MT Jobs	http://www.mtjobs.com	A job board devoted to employment for medical transcriptionists.
OR Live	http://www.orlive.com/	A site featuring live broadcasts of actual surgeries as well as a library of videos from prior procedures, demonstrations of medical equipment, and answers to e-mail questions during procedures. The site also contains archives of forum discussion of medical issues as well as current medical news.
RX List	http://fdb.rxlist.com/drugs/	A comprehensive listing of drugs listed by both generic and brand names.
The Agape Center	http://theagapecenter.com/Hospitals/index.htm	A hospital locator in any state. Select name of state, then browse hospital listings for that state.
UCLA Medical School	http://www.wilkes.med.ucla.edu/intro.html	The "Auscultation Assistant" site enables students to click on the heart illustration to view a list containing a variety of heart sounds along with medical terminology associated with each.
U-Compare	http://www.ucomparehealthcare.com/	A physician locator in any state. Search by name or specialty using the "browse" links in the middle of the page.
Wound Care Information Network	http://www.medicaledu.com/default.htm	A site devoted to information and terminology about wound care.

Institute for Safe Medication Practices

ISMP's List of *Error-Prone Abbreviations*, Symbols, and *Dose Designations*

The abbreviations, symbols, and dose designations found in this table have been reported to ISMP through the ISMP National Medication Errors Reporting Program (ISMP MERP) as being frequently misinterpreted and involved in harmful medication errors. They should **NEVER** be used when communicating medical information. This includes internal communications, telephone/verbal prescriptions, computer-generated labels, labels for drug storage bins, medication administration records, as well as pharmacy and prescriber computer order entry screens.

Abbreviations	Intended Meaning	Misinterpretation	Correction
μg	Microgram	Mistaken as "mg"	Use "mcg"
AD, AS, AU	Right ear, left ear, each ear	Mistaken as OD, OS, OU (right eye, left eye, each eye)	Use "right ear," "left ear," or "each ear"
OD, OS, OU	Right eye, left eye, each eye	Mistaken as AD, AS, AU (right ear, left ear, each ear)	Use "right eye," "left eye," or "each eye"
BT	Bedtime	Mistaken as "BID" (twice daily)	Use "bedtime"
cc	Cubic centimeters	Mistaken as "u" (units)	Use "mL"
D/C	Discharge or discontinue	Premature discontinuation of medications if D/C (intended to mean "discharge") has been misinterpreted as "discontinued" when followed by a list of discharge medications	Use "discharge" and "discontinue"
IJ	Injection	Mistaken as "IV" or "intrajugular"	Use "injection"
IN	Intranasal	Mistaken as "IM" or "IV"	Use "intranasal" or "NAS"
HS	Half-strength	Mistaken as bedtime	Use "half-strength" or "bedtime"
hs	At bedtime, hours of sleep	Mistaken as half-strength	
IU**	International unit	Mistaken as IV (intravenous) or 10 (ten)	Use "units"
o.d. or OD	Once daily	Mistaken as "right eye" (OD-oculus dexter), leading to oral liquid medications administered in the eye	Use "daily"
OJ	Orange juice	Mistaken as OD or OS (right or left eye); drugs meant to be diluted in orange juice may be given in the eye	Use "orange juice"
Per os	By mouth, orally	The "os" can be mistaken as "left eye" (OS-oculus sinister)	Use "PO," "by mouth," or "orally"
q.d. or QD**	Every day	Mistaken as q.i.d., especially if the period after the "q" or the tail of the "q" is misunderstood as an "i"	Use "daily"
qhs	Nightly at bedtime	Mistaken as "qhr" or every hour	Use "nightly"
qn	Nightly or at bedtime	Mistaken as "qh" (every hour)	Use "nightly" or "at bedtime"
q.o.d. or QOD**	Every other day	Mistaken as "q.d." (daily) or "q.i.d. (four times daily) if the "o" is poorly written	Use "every other day"
q1d	Daily	Mistaken as q.i.d. (four times daily)	Use "daily"
q6PM, etc.	Every evening at 6 PM	Mistaken as every 6 hours	Use "daily at 6 PM" or "6 PM daily"
SC, SQ, sub q	Subcutaneous	SC mistaken as SL (sublingual); SQ mistaken as "5 every;" the "q" in "sub q" has been mistaken as "every" (e.g., a heparin dose ordered "sub q 2 hours before surgery" misunderstood as every 2 hours before surgery)	Use "subcut" or "subcutaneously"
ss	Sliding scale (insulin) or ½ (apothecary)	Mistaken as "55"	Spell out "sliding scale;" use "one-half" or "½"
SSRI	Sliding scale regular insulin	Mistaken as selective-serotonin reuptake inhibitor	Spell out "sliding scale (insulin)"
SSI	Sliding scale insulin	Mistaken as Strong Solution of Iodine (Lugol's)	
i/d	One daily	Mistaken as "tid"	Use "1 daily"
TIW or tiw	3 times a week	Mistaken as "3 times a day" or "twice in a week"	Use "3 times weekly"
U or u**	Unit	Mistaken as the number 0 or 4, causing a 10-fold overdose or greater (e.g., 4U seen as "40" or 4u seen as "44"); mistaken as "cc" so dose given in volume instead of units (e.g., 4u seen as 4cc)	Use "unit"
UD	As directed ("ut dictum")	Mistaken as unit dose (e.g., diltiazem 125 mg IV infusion "UD" misinterpreted as meaning to give the entire infusion as a unit [bolus] dose)	Use "as directed"
Dose Designations and Other Information	Intended Meaning	Misinterpretation	Correction
Trailing zero after decimal point (e.g., 1.0 mg)**	1 mg	Mistaken as 10 mg if the decimal point is not seen	Do not use trailing zeros for doses expressed in whole numbers
"Naked" decimal point (e.g., .5 mg)**	0.5 mg	Mistaken as 5 mg if the decimal point is not seen	Use zero before a decimal point when the dose is less than a whole unit
Abbreviations such as mg. or mL. with a period following the abbreviation	mg mL	The period is unnecessary and could be mistaken as the number 1 if written poorly	Use mg, mL, etc. without a terminal period

Institute for Safe Medication Practices

ISMP's **List of** *Error-Prone Abbreviations, Symbols,* **and** *Dose Designations* (continued)

Dose Designations and Other Information	Intended Meaning	Misinterpretation	Correction
Drug name and dose run together (especially problematic for drug names that end in "l" such as Inderal40 mg; Tegretol300 mg)	Inderal 40 mg Tegretol 300 mg	Mistaken as Inderal 140 mg Mistaken as Tegretol 1300 mg	Place adequate space between the drug name, dose, and unit of measure
Numerical dose and unit of measure run together (e.g., 10mg, 100mL)	10 mg 100 mL	The "m" is sometimes mistaken as a zero or two zeros, risking a 10- to 100-fold overdose	Place adequate space between the dose and unit of measure
Large doses without properly placed commas (e.g., 100000 units; 1000000 units)	100,000 units 1,000,000 units	100000 has been mistaken as 10,000 or 1,000,000; 1000000 has been mistaken as 100,000	Use commas for dosing units at or above 1,000, or use words such as 100 "thousand" or 1 "million" to improve readability

Drug Name Abbreviations	Intended Meaning	Misinterpretation	Correction
To avoid confusion, do not abbreviate drug names when communicating medical information. Examples of drug name abbreviations involved in medication errors include:			
APAP	acetaminophen	Not recognized as acetaminophen	Use complete drug name
ARA A	vidarabine	Mistaken as cytarabine (ARA C)	Use complete drug name
AZT	zidovudine (Retrovir)	Mistaken as azathioprine or aztreonam	Use complete drug name
CPZ	Compazine (prochlorperazine)	Mistaken as chlorpromazine	Use complete drug name
DPT	Demerol-Phenergan-Thorazine	Mistaken as diphtheria-pertussis-tetanus (vaccine)	Use complete drug name
DTO	Diluted tincture of opium, or deodorized tincture of opium (Paregoric)	Mistaken as tincture of opium	Use complete drug name
HCl	hydrochloric acid or hydrochloride	Mistaken as potassium chloride (The "H" is misinterpreted as "K")	Use complete drug name unless expressed as a salt of a drug
HCT	hydrocortisone	Mistaken as hydrochlorothiazide	Use complete drug name
HCTZ	hydrochlorothiazide	Mistaken as hydrocortisone (seen as HCT250 mg)	Use complete drug name
MgSO4**	magnesium sulfate	Mistaken as morphine sulfate	Use complete drug name
MS, MSO4**	morphine sulfate	Mistaken as magnesium sulfate	Use complete drug name
MTX	methotrexate	Mistaken as mitoxantrone	Use complete drug name
PCA	procainamide	Mistaken as patient controlled analgesia	Use complete drug name
PTU	propylthiouracil	Mistaken as mercaptopurine	Use complete drug name
T3	Tylenol with codeine No. 3	Mistaken as liothyronine	Use complete drug name
TAC	triamcinolone	Mistaken as tetracaine, Adrenalin, cocaine	Use complete drug name
TNK	TNKase	Mistaken as "TPA"	Use complete drug name
ZnSO4	zinc sulfate	Mistaken as morphine sulfate	Use complete drug name

Stemmed Drug Names	Intended Meaning	Misinterpretation	Correction
"Nitro" drip	nitroglycerin infusion	Mistaken as sodium nitroprusside infusion	Use complete drug name
"Norflox"	norfloxacin	Mistaken as Norflex	Use complete drug name
"IV Vanc"	intravenous vancomycin	Mistaken as Invanz	Use complete drug name

Symbols	Intended Meaning	Misinterpretation	Correction
ℨ ℔	Dram Minim	Symbol for dram mistaken as "3" Symbol for minim mistaken as "mL"	Use the metric system
x3d	For three days	Mistaken as "3 doses"	Use "for three days"
> and <	Greater than and less than	Mistaken as opposite of intended; mistakenly use incorrect symbol; "< 10" mistaken as "40"	Use "greater than" or "less than"
/ (slash mark)	Separates two doses or indicates "per"	Mistaken as the number 1 (e.g., "25 units/10 units" misread as "25 units and 110" units)	Use "per" rather than a slash mark to separate doses
@	At	Mistaken as "2"	Use "at"
&	And	Mistaken as "2"	Use "and"
+	Plus or and	Mistaken as "4"	Use "and"
°	Hour	Mistaken as a zero (e.g., q2° seen as q 20)	Use "hr," "h," or "hour"
Ø or ⦰	zero, null sign	Mistaken as numerals 4, 6, 8, and 9	Use 0 or zero, or describe intent using whole words

**These abbreviations are included on The Joint Commission's "minimum list" of dangerous abbreviations, acronyms, and symbols that must be included on an organization's "Do Not Use" list, effective January 1, 2004. Visit www.jointcommission.org for more information about this Joint Commission requirement.

ISMP
INSTITUTE FOR SAFE MEDICATION PRACTICES
www.ismp.org

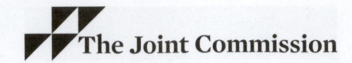

The Joint Commission

Official "Do Not Use" List[1]

Do Not Use	Potential Problem	Use Instead
U (unit)	Mistaken for "0" (zero), the number "4" (four) or "cc"	Write "unit"
IU (International Unit)	Mistaken for IV (intravenous) or the number 10 (ten)	Write "International Unit"
Q.D., QD, q.d., qd (daily)	Mistaken for each other	Write "daily"
Q.O.D., QOD, q.o.d, qod (every other day)	Period after the Q mistaken for "I" and the "O" mistaken for "I"	Write "every other day"
Trailing zero (X.0 mg)* Lack of leading zero (.X mg)	Decimal point is missed	Write X mg Write 0.X mg
MS	Can mean morphine sulfate or magnesium sulfate	Write "morphine sulfate" Write "magnesium sulfate"
MSO_4 and $MgSO_4$	Confused for one another	

[1] Applies to all orders and all medication-related documentation that is handwritten (including free-text computer entry) or on pre-printed forms.

*Exception: A "trailing zero" may be used only where required to demonstrate the level of precision of the value being reported, such as for laboratory results, imaging studies that report size of lesions, or catheter/tube sizes. It may not be used in medication orders or other medication-related documentation.

Additional Abbreviations, Acronyms and Symbols
(For possible future inclusion in the Official "Do Not Use" List)

Do Not Use	Potential Problem	Use Instead
> (greater than) < (less than)	Misinterpreted as the number "7" (seven) or the letter "L" Confused for one another	Write "greater than" Write "less than"
Abbreviations for drug names	Misinterpreted due to similar abbreviations for multiple drugs	Write drug names in full
Apothecary units	Unfamiliar to many practitioners Confused with metric units	Use metric units
@	Mistaken for the number "2" (two)	Write "at"
cc	Mistaken for U (units) when poorly written	Write "mL" or "ml" or "milliliters" ("mL" is preferred)
µg	Mistaken for mg (milligrams) resulting in one thousand-fold overdose	Write "mcg" or "micrograms"

APPENDIX B

Normal Laboratory Values and Commonly Used Metric System Units and Symbols

NORMAL LABORATORY VALUES

HEMATOLOGY TESTS

Name of Test	Normal Range
Complete Blood Count	
Erythrocyte sedimentation rate (Westergren)	
Female	0–30 mm/h
Male	0–20 mm/h
Hematocrit (Hct)	
Female	36–46%
Male	42–52%
Hemoglobin (Hgb)	
Female	12–16 g/dL
Male	14–17 g/dL
Mean corpuscular hemoglobin (MCH)	27–33 pg/cell
Mean corpuscular volume (MCV)	80–97.6 mcm^3
Platelet count	100,000 – 450,000/mm^3
Red blood cells (RBC) (x 10^6 mL)	
Female	4.0–4.9
Male	4.5–5.5
Red cell distribution width (RDW)	<14.5
Reticulocyte count	0.5–2.5%
White blood cell count (WBC)	4.5–11
White blood cell differential	
Segmented neutrophils	40–80%
Band neutrophils	3–5%
Basophils	0–0.2%
Eosinophils	0–5%

Reprinted with permission from the Medical Council of Canada (MCC).

(Continues)

Name of Test	Normal Range
Lymphocytes	25−35%
Monocytes	2−10%
Other Blood and Chemistry Tests:	
Albumin	3.5−4.2%
Alkaline phosphatase	33−131 IU/L
Alanine (ALT; SGPT)	<35 IU/L
Aspartate (AST; SGOT)	<35 IU/L
Amylase	53−123 U/L
Bicarbonate	22−29 mEq/L
Bilirubin	
Direct Bilirubin	0−0.4 mg/dL
Total Bilirubin	1.0−1.8 mg/dL
Calcium	
Ionized	2.24−2.46 mEq/dL
Total	8.8−10.3 mg/dL
Chloride	95−107 mEq/dL
Cholesterol	<200 mg/dL
Cortisol	6−23 mcg/dL
Creatine kinase (total CK; CPK)	60−400 IU/L
Creatine kinase myocardial band (CK−MB)	0−3 ng/mL
Creatinine	0.5−4.4
Ferritin	13−300 ng/mL
Folate	3.6−20 ng/dL
Glucose fasting	60−110
Hemoglobin A_1C	6−8
High density lipoprotein (HDL cholesterol)	30−70 mg/dL
Iron	65−150 mcg/dL
Lactic acid	0.7−2.1 mEq/dL
Lactic dehydrogenase (LDH)	56−194 IU/L
Low density lipoprotein (LDL cholesterol)	65−180 mg/dL
Lipase	10−150 IU/L
Magnesium	1.6−2.4 mEq/dL
Osmolality	289−308
Phosphorus	2.5−4.5 mEq/dL
Potassium	3.5−5.2 mEq/dL
Prostate Specific Antigen (PSA)	0−4 ng/mL
Protein (total)	6.0−8.4 g/dL
Sodium	135−147 mEq/dL
Thyroid-stimulating hormone (sensitive)	0.25−4.30

Name of Test	Normal Range
T3 (free)	2.3−4.2 pg/mL
T4 (free)	0.5−2.1 ng/dL
Total iron binding capacity (TIBC)	250−420 mcg/dL
Triglycerides	45−155 mg/dL
Troponin	<0.4 ng/mL
Urea nitrogen (BUN)	7−20 mg/dL
Uric acid	
Female	2.0−7.0 ng/mL
Male	2.1−8.5 ng/mL
Coagulation Studies	
Bleeding time	<9 minutes
International Normalized Ratio (INR)	0.9−1.2
Partial thromboplastin time (PTT)	28−38 seconds
Prothrombin time (PT) ("pro time")	10−13 seconds

Reprinted with permission from the Medical Council of Canada (MCC).

URINALYSIS

Name of Test	Normal Range
Calcium	<7.3 mmol/day
Chloride	110−250 mmol/day
Cortisol	10−100 mcg/24h
Creatinine	6.2−17.7 mmol/day
Osmolality	100−1200 mOsm/kg
Potassium	25−120 mmol/day
Protein	<0.15 g/day
Sodium	25−260 mmol/day
Specific Gravity	1.001−1.030

Reprinted with permission from the Medical Council of Canada (MCC).

ARTERIAL BLOOD GAS

Name of Test	Normal Values
pH	7.35−7.45
PaO_2	80−100
$PaCO_2$	35−45
HCO_3 (bicarbonate)	19−25
SaO_2 (saturation)	95−99%

Reprinted with permission from the Medical Council of Canada (MCC).

PULMONARY FUNCTION TESTING

FVC	FEV1	FEV1 / FVC
Normal: 80–100% of predicted	**Normal:** 80–100% of predicted	**Normal:** 80–100% of predicted
Decreased:	**Decreased:**	**Decreased:**
Mild: 65–80% of predicted	Mild: 65–80% of predicted	Mild: 65–80% of predicted
Mod: 50–65% of predicted	Mod: 50–65% of predicted	Mod: 50–65% of predicted
Severe: < 50% of predicted	Severe: < 50% of predicted	Severe: < 50% of predicted

Reprinted with permission from the Medical Council of Canada (MCC).

COMMONLY USED METRIC SYSTEM UNITS AND SYMBOLS

Quantity Measured	Unit	Symbol	Relationship		
Area	square meter	m^2			
	hectare	ha	1 ha	=	10 000 m^2
	square kilometer	km^2	1 km^2	=	100 ha
Density	kilogram per cubic meter	kg/m^3			
Energy	kilojoule	kJ			
	megajoule	MJ	1 MJ	=	1000 kJ
	kilowatt hour	kW·h	1 kW·h	=	3.6 MJ
Electric current	ampere	A			
Force	newton	N			
Length, width, distance, thickness, girth, etc.	millimeter	mm	10 mm	=	1 cm
	centimeter	cm	100 cm	=	1 m
	meter	m			
	kilometer	km	1 km	=	1000 m
Mass ("weight")	milligram	mg	1000 mg	=	1 g
	gram	g			
	kilogram	kg	1 kg	=	1000 g
	metric ton	t	1 t	=	1000 kg
Pressure, stress	kilopascal	kPa			
Power	watt	W			
	kilowatt	kW	1 kW	=	1000 W
Speed, velocity	meter per second	m/s			
	kilometer per hour	km/h	1 km/h	=	0.278 m/s
Temperature	degree Celsius	°C			
Time	second	s			
Volume	milliliter	mL	1000 mL	=	1 L
	cubic centimeter	cm^3	1 cm^3	=	1 mL
	liter	L	1000 L	=	1 m^3
	cubic meter	m^3			

Reprinted with permission from the U.S. Metric Association. For more information, visit http://www.metric.org.

2-D ECHOCARDIOGRAM

1. Left ventricle is mildly dilated, with normal left ventricular wall thickness. There is mild to moderate left ventricular systolic dysfunction. There is paradoxical septal motion, consistent with the postoperative state. The estimated ejection fraction is approximately 40%.
2. The right ventricle is mildly dilated.
3. There is mild thickening of the anterior leaflet of the mitral valve, with normal leaflet mobility. There is no evidence of mitral valve prolapse. There is mild mitral regurgitation.
4. There is a normally functioning homograft valve in the aortic position. There is no aortic insufficiency. There are no identifiable vegetations on the aortic valve prosthesis.
5. The tricuspid valve is morphologically normal. There is a trivial degree of tricuspid regurgitation.
6. There is no pulmonic insufficiency.
7. The left atrium is mildy to moderately dilated.
8. There is no significant pericardial effusion.
9. The right atrium is normal.
10. The aorta is normal.
11. Doppler: mitral valve 1 m/s aortic valve 1.3 m/s tricuspid valve 0.5 m/s. Pulmonary valve 0.6 m/s.

IMPRESSION:

1. Left ventricular chamber size is increased, with normal wall thickness. There is paradoxical septal movement, consistent with a postoperative state.
2. There is a normal functioning homograft noted in the aortic position. There is no evidence of perivalvular leak or vegetations.
3. Mild mitral regurgitation and trivial tricuspid regurgitation.

CLINIC NOTE

HISTORY OF PRESENT ILLNESS: Patient reports a mass in the left side of his neck, which has been present over 3 months. The patient is a 55-year-old male and notes that the mass has gradually increased in size over the past 3 months. He states the mass is approximately the size of a marble. The mass is not tender and is completely asymptomatic. He denies a history of smoking or alcohol abuse. He denies weight loss, hemoptysis, sore throat, or dysphasia. He denies shortness of breath. He denies any recent infection.

PAST MEDICAL HISTORY: Coronary artery disease and hypertension, for which he takes digoxin and Lasix.

ALLERGIES: He is not allergic to any medications.

PHYSICAL EXAMINATION: The ears are within normal limits. The nose reveals inflamed mucosa, with no masses or purulence. The oropharynx and oral cavity are without masses or lesions. There are no palpable masses in the oropharynx, oral cavity, or base of tongue. Clear fluid is expressed from Stensen's and Wharton's ducts bilaterally. The nasopharynx, hypopharynx, and larynx are within normal limits. The neck exam reveals a 2 cm firm mass in the tail of the left parotid gland. The remainder of the neck is without masses or nodes. Facial motor function is symmetrical and intact bilaterally.

IMPRESSION: In summary, the patient has a mass in the tail of the left parotid gland.

PLAN: I have explained to the patient that further evaluation is necessary. I have recommended that he undergo a fine-needle aspiration of the left parotid mass, and this will be scheduled. This procedure will be performed under local anesthesia, and the nature, course, and complications, including bleeding, infection, and failure to make the diagnosis, were explained, and consent was obtained. In addition, I have recommended that he have a CT scan of the neck with contrast to evaluate the location and nature of the mass in the left parotid gland. He will bring the CT scan results with him to his appointment for the needle aspiration.

CONSULTATION

REASON FOR CONSULTATION: Abnormal liver enzymes.

HISTORY OF PRESENT ILLNESS: This is a 60-year-old female with a history of chronic paranoid schizophrenia admitted to the hospital for high fever, cough, yellow phlegm, and chest x-ray consistent with pneumonia. The patient was treated with Rocephin and had improvement. The temperature on admission was 101 degrees, peaking at 102 degrees, and then gradually defervesced. The SMAC panel revealed abnormal liver enzymes, and I was asked to see the patient.

On questioning, the patient was an extremely poor historian. She has marked lability of affect and is not able to carry on an appropriate conversation due to spontaneous laughing and crying spells. The patient is also very tangential and thus it is not possible to get a good history from. Therefore, the bulk of her history is obtained from the chart.

PAST MEDICAL HISTORY: Remarkable for schizophrenia.

CURRENT MEDICATIONS:
1. Haldol.
2. Cogentin.
3. Lithium.
4. Dilantin.
5. Klonopin.

FAMILY HISTORY: Please see the chart.

SOCIAL HISTORY: Please see the chart.

REVIEW OF SYSTEMS: Please see the chart.

PHYSICAL EXAMINATION:

GENERAL: This is an elderly patient who has a somewhat hirsute facies.

VITAL SIGNS: On arrival, the temperature was 101 degrees, pulse 100, respirations 26, and blood pressure 118/72.

HEENT: Normocephalic, pupils equal and reactive to light, no frank icterus. The patient has a waxy pallor to her entire facies.

NECK: Supple, no lymphadenopathy or jugular venous distention.

HEART: The point of maximum impulse is the 5th interspace. S1 and S2 are regular, no gallop or murmur.

CHEST: Symmetrical, harsh fascicular breath sounds, occasional rales.

ABDOMEN: Soft, well-healed scar from previous surgery present in the right lower quadrant. No definite tenderness appreciated in any quadrant, no definite masses, bowel sounds absent.

EXTREMITIES: No clubbing, edema, or calf tenderness.

NEUROLOGIC: The patient is awake, tangential, and without obvious cranial nerve deficit. Sensory and motor systems appear physiologic.

LABORATORY DATA: Hemoglobin 12, hematocrit 35.8, white count 6,400, with normal indices of 68 segs, 5 bands, 11 eosinophils, 6 monos and 10 lymphs. BUN and creatinine are unremarkable. Electrolytes are within normal limits. Blood sugar is 77, GGT abnormal at 328. Other values included SGPT 107, SGOT 60, alkaline phosphatase 175, LDH 165, total bilirubin 0.4, total protein 7.4, albumin low at 2.5, and globulin high at 4.9. The patient had an abdominal ultrasound, which revealed cholelithiasis. A hepatitis panel was recommended and this revealed hepatitis B surface antigen negative.

IMPRESSION: A 60-year-old female with a history of schizophrenia, pneumonia, and abnormal liver enzymes. The drugs to be particularly concerned about would be Dilantin, which can cause hepatocellular damage, and other phenothiazine-type medications, in other words, Haldol. Other possibilities could include passage of a stone from the cholelithiasis. Lastly, a transpneumonitis secondary to the pneumonia; however, the patient seems to be holding the abnormal liver enzymes despite clinical improvement in this pneumonia.

PLAN: At this point, I would recommend monitoring of the liver enzymes and if there is further elevation, a liver biopsy should be done or withdrawal from the Dilantin medication. We could certainly replace the Dilantin with another antiseizure medication.

DISCHARGE SUMMARY

DISCHARGE DIAGNOSES:

1. Lymphadenitis, resolving.
2. Fever thought secondary to infection.

PROCEDURES PERFORMED: Incision and drainage of left subauricular fluctuant abscess.

HISTORY OF PRESENT ILLNESS: The patient is a healthy 6-month-old child who was well until approximately 4 days prior to admission when she was noted to have a subauricular swelling on a routine check-up. At that time, the mother denied any fevers, dietary problems, fussiness, etc. The patient was given dicloxacillin for 2 days, but she refused to take any more. For this reason, the mother brought the child to the emergency room.

PHYSICAL EXAMINATION: On physical examination, the child was a happy, playful child in no acute distress. The examination was remarkable for a firm and movable 2.5 × 3 cm node, which was underneath the left ear and which was slightly warm and tender.

LABORATORY DATA: White count 14,300 and negative blood cultures from the emergency room visit.

HOSPITAL COURSE: The patient was admitted to the floor with the diagnosis of left subauricular lymphadenitis and was started on intravenous Kefzol. The patient's swelling became more localized and fluctuant by the 4th day in the hospital, and it was incised and drained without difficulty. The intravenous Kefzol was continued for an 8-day course. The wound was packed with gauze after the incision and drainage, and healed very nicely. The patient remained fairly afebrile during her hospital course, with her temperature barely reaching to 100.4 degrees. On hospital day #8, the patient was ready for discharge and will be continued on p.o. medications at home. The wound does not require further packing, as it is a very small abscess pocket.

DISPOSITION: The patient is discharged to home.

DISCHARGE MEDICATIONS: Dicloxacillin 2 teaspoonfuls p.o. at bedtime for 4 days.

DISCHARGE INSTRUCTIONS:

1. The patient is to follow up in the office in 1 week.
2. The parents were instructed to bring the child to the emergency room for any increase in swelling, fever, or redness in the subauricular area.

HISTORY AND PHYSICAL EXAMINATION

HISTORY OF PRESENT ILLNESS: This is the initial visit of this very pleasant 73-year-old female who states that she developed atrial fibrillation 5 years ago. She has seen another cardiologist for this and now wishes to switch cardiologists. She has been taking Quinaglute since that time and Calan, but has been complaining of dry mouth, diarrhea, loss of energy, and tooth pain. As of this past month she has weaned herself off these medications, and her symptoms immediately improved. During that time period, she had been taking quinidine on a p.r.n.-type basis, prescribed by herself only.

She complains of occasional irregular heartbeat and skipping. She denies any syncope or lightheadedness. She also complains of chest pressure, which occurs once a week and lasts for approximately 1 hour. It seems to occur with increased activity. Her last exercise treadmill test was approximately 1 year ago.

CORONARY RISK FACTORS: Negative hypertension, negative diabetes, negative smoking, unknown cholesterol status.

CURRENT MEDICATIONS:
1. Quinaglute 324 mg t.i.d.
2. Calan 80 mg.

ALLERGIES: HORSE SERUM.

PAST SURGICAL HISTORY:
1. Right upper lobe removal secondary to lung cancer.
2. Ovarian cyst removal.

PAST MEDICAL HISTORY: Atrial fibrillation.

SOCIAL HISTORY: She is married. She denies the use of ethanol or cigarettes. She drinks approximately 2 cups of coffee per day.

REVIEW OF SYSTEMS: Noncontributory.

FAMILY HISTORY: Noncontributory.

PHYSICAL EXAMINATION:

GENERAL: Alert, oriented, in no acute distress.

VITAL SIGNS: Blood pressure is 134/80, heart rate is 75.

NECK: Supple, without jugular venous distention or bruits.

LUNGS: Clear, without wheezing, rhonchi, or rales.

HEART: Regular rate and rhythm, without murmurs, gallops, or rubs. There is an occasional extrasystole noted.

ABDOMEN: Soft, nontender, without mass or organomegaly.

EXTREMITIES: Without edema.

LABORATORY DATA: EKG: PR interval 0.18. QRS interval 0.06. Axis −35 degrees.

Interpretation: Sinus rhythm, rate of 70. Frequent PACs, prominent U waves.

IMPRESSION AND PLAN:

1. History of atrial fibrillation. This patient gives a history of atrial fibrillation, which she has been treated with Coumadin for in the past. At the present time she is in sinus rhythm, with frequent PACs. The possibility of paroxysmal atrial fibrillation is, of course, present in her. Because she does complain of frequent palpitations, we will put a 24-hour Holter monitor on her to see if we can capture these episodes. I will request an EKG and records from her previous physician as well. I have also advised her to completely stop her quinidine, as quinidine has been found to have increased mortality in people treated with atrial fibrillation. I have asked her to begin aspirin 81 mg once a day. If she does, in fact, have paroxysmal atrial fibrillation, I feel the patient should be anticoagulated fully with Coumadin.

2. Chest discomfort. The patient complains of exertional chest discomfort. I will plan to do an exercise thallium stress test on her to help exclude ischemia. I will have her follow up following the stress test and Holter results.

A 24-HOUR HOLTER MONITOR

Holter monitoring performed for 24 hours. Predominant rhythm is sinus. The average heartbeat is 69 beats per minute. Range is 44 to 104 beats per minute. There are frequent PVCs noted, averaging 1193 per hour. There are frequent ventricular couplets noted. There are 4 three-beat ones of nonsustained ventricular tachycardia noted. There are no sustained runs of ventricular tachycardia.

There is an occasional PAC noted. There are 3 runs of nonsustained supraventricular tachycardia (the longest one 11 beats, maximal heart rate 153). There were no sustained runs of supraventricular tachycardia.

There were no prolonged sinus pauses noted. There was no evidence of high-degree AV block.

Maximal ST depression is 1.8 mm. The significance of this is unclear.

Patient noted throbbing in her neck several times in her diary and was noted to be in the sinus rhythm with a heart rate of between 70 and 77, with an occasional PVC. She also noted dyspnea and was noted to be in sinus rhythm with a heart rate of 87, with an occasional PVC. Patient also recorded shortness of breath and lightheadedness and was noted to be in sinus rhythm, with an occasional PVC and a regular heart rate of 78.

CONCLUSION: Abnormal Holter, revealing frequent and complex ventricular ectopy, nonsustained ventricular tachycardia, and nonsustained supraventricular tachycardia. ST depressions of unknown significance.

IMAGING STUDY

NOTE TO STUDENT: AN "IMAGING STUDY" CAN BE AN X-RAY, CT SCAN, MRI, OR OTHER IMAGING STUDY.

NAME OF TEST: Computerized tomography of the abdomen and pelvis.

INDICATION: Blood per rectum.

TECHNIQUE: Axial CT images were obtained from the dome of the liver through the symphysis pubis. Oral, rectal, and intravenous contrasts were given.

FINDINGS: There is a 2×2.4 cm, round, fluid-attenuation lesion within the left liver lobe, lateral segment, consistent with a simple cyst. The gallbladder, spleen, pancreas, and adrenals are within normal limits. The left kidney is somewhat malrotated, normal variant.

There is a moderate amount of food within the stomach. No gastrointestinal lesions are seen.

There is no aortic aneurysm. No adenopathy is noted. Images through the patient's pelvis demonstrate a normal-appearing bladder and uterus.

IMPRESSION: Liver cyst. Otherwise within normal limits. Given the history of blood per rectum, consideration for further evaluation with either a barium enema or endoscopy should be given.

LETTER

Date

Dr. Wang Hong
100 North Bay Avenue
Nashville, TN 37202

Re: Patient: Ernesto Tovar

Dear Dr. Hong:

I had the opportunity to see Mr. Tovar in consultation to discuss his opportunity for renal transplantation. The patient came alone to consultation. As you know, Mr. Tovar is a 67-year-old Hispanic male who has end-stage renal disease secondary to diabetes mellitus and hypertension. He is on hemodialysis every Monday, Wednesday, and Friday.

During our 30-minute consultation, I reviewed available results of medical tests performed today and explained in detail the nature of preoperative phase and postoperative phase of renal transplantation. Considerable time was spent with him regarding the need for chronic long-term immunosuppression and its risks. I would recommend a cadaveric renal transplantation. Considering his age and the long waiting time, which currently exceeds 5 years in the State of Tennessee, I would also recommend to inquire about a living donor and to see whether his son would be a suitable candidate.

Thank you for the opportunity to be a part of this patient's care and for your support of the transplant activities at University of Illinois. If you have any questions regarding this patient, please do not hesitate to call me directly.

Sincerely,

Joseph Anderson, MD

JA/xx

OPERATIVE REPORT 1

PATIENT: William Jones

DATE OF OPERATION: (Current date)

OPERATING SURGEON: George Smith, MD

ASSISTANT: William Harris, MD

ANESTHESIA: General.

ANESTHESIOLOGIST: James Montgomery, MD

PREOPERATIVE DIAGNOSIS: Diabetic gangrene of the left foot.

POSTOPERATIVE DIAGNOSIS: Diabetic gangrene of the left foot.

OPERATION PERFORMED: Below-knee amputation of the left lower extremity.

OPERATIVE TECHNIQUE: The patient was prepped and draped in a routine manner under general anesthesia with endotracheal intubation. He had been given Cefotan antibiotic 2 g intravenously prior to incision.

A skin incision was made approximately 3 fingerbreadths below the tibial tuberosity on the left side. Dissection was carried circumferentially around the leg at that point, dividing the subcutaneous tissue. Bleeders were clamped and tied with 2-0 chromic ligature. Muscle compartments and fascias were divided with sharp dissection. Anteriorly, the dissection was carried down to the periosteum covering the tibia. At that point, using blunt and sharp dissection, the periosteum was elevated from the anterior surface of the tibia with a periosteal elevator. The anterior compartment muscles were then divided with sharp dissection, bleeders again being clamped and tied with 2-0 chromic or 0 Vicryl suture ligatures. A Crile clamp was then passed behind the tibia, and a Gigli saw was brought posterior to the bone. The Gigli saw was then used to transect the bone at that point. The fibula was then identified and exposed proximal to the tibial division. Using a bone cutter, the tibia was divided approximately one-half inch above the tibial transection. A large amputation knife was then used to divide the muscles on the posterior compartment. The larger vessel and nerve groups were identified, cross clamped and divided, and tied with 2-0 Vicryl suture ligature.

The incision was then closed, after hemostasis was complete and the dissection area had been thoroughly irrigated with warm saline solution, by approximating the anterior and posterior muscle fascia coverings with interrupted 2-0 chromic suture. A quarter-inch Penrose drain placed under the fascial closure was brought out medially and laterally via the corners of the skin incision. The skin was then closed with interrupted 4-0 nylon mattress suture. An Adaptic 4 × 4 ABD Kerlix dressing was then applied.

The patient tolerated the procedure well. Blood loss was estimated at approximately 100 mL. He left the operating room in stable condition.

OPERATIVE REPORT 2

PREOPERATIVE DIAGNOSIS: Cataract, left eye.

POSTOPERATIVE DIAGNOSIS: Cataract, left eye.

PROCEDURE: Extracapsular cataract extraction with implantation of a Viscolens posterior chamber intraocular lens.

ANESTHESIA: Retrobulbar and van lint periorbital block with standby anesthesia monitoring.

PROCEDURE IN DETAIL: Following a discussion with the anesthesiologist, the patient was brought to the operating suite, where several drops of 0.5% proparacaine were instilled into the left palpebral fissure. A 50-50 mixture of 2% lidocaine and 0.5% bupivacaine with 75 units of Wydase was carefully injected retrobulbarly by the surgeon. Using the same solution, 3 mL of additional periorbital van lint anesthesia was administered. The eye was then gently massaged for 1 minute.

The patient was then prepped and draped in the usual sterile fashion. A 6-0 Vicryl suture was used for traction at the inferior corneal limbus through the superior rectus tendons. A fornix-based conjunctival flap was then created superiorly using Westcott scissors. Hemostasis was achieved using wet-field cautery forceps. A 2 mm corneal groove was made with a #69 Beaver blade. OcuCoat viscoelastic was injected into the anterior chamber. A bent 25-gauge disposable needle, which was attached to a balanced salt infusion, was used to incise the lens capsule superiorly. Using the same needle, the lens nucleus was engaged, gently rotated, and hydrodissected from the adjacent peripheral cortex. Curved corneal scissors were used to complete the corneal resection which was then secured with 2 preplaced 10-0 nylon sutures. The lens nucleus was manually expressed, avoiding contact with the corneal endothelium as much as possible. The preplaced sutures were tied tightly with bow knots.

The Simcoe cannula was then inserted through the incision in the lens capsule and the lens cortex was aspirated with manual suction. Viscoelastic material was injected to distend the lens capsule and to maintain the anterior chamber. An Ioptex UVB 308-10 6.5 mm optic posterior chamber intraocular lens was implanted into the ciliary sulcus.

The capsulotomy was completed by tearing the inferior portion of the capsule superiorly and removing the excised anterior capsule with Utrata forceps. The viscoelastic was aspirated from the anterior chamber with the Simcoe cannula.

Pilocarpine was used to constrict the pupil. Additional 10-0 nylon interrupted sutures were used to close the corneal incision. The wound was inspected and found to be watertight. Garamycin 20 mg and 2 mg of Decadron were injected subconjunctivally. The 6-0 Vicryl traction suture was removed and TobraDex ointment was instilled into the palpebral fissure. A sterile pad and protective shield were applied to the left eye.

The patient left the operating room in good condition and was given a followup appointment.

CLINIC NOTE

NOTE TO STUDENT: THIS CLINIC NOTE USES ONE FORM OF THE "SOAP" FORMAT.

S: A 23-month-old brought in by Mother because of tugging at the ears. The mother was concerned that she might have an ear infection. Incidentally, she continues to be breastfed at 23 months of age.

O: The physical examination showed that the tympanic membranes were slightly retracted, but there were no air-fluid levels or inflammation. The rest of the physical examination was negative.

A: More time was spent talking about the baby's persistence in breastfeeding as the returns on that were felt to be diminishing and an effort was made diplomatically to convince the mother to begin to wean the baby.

P: The plan was medically to give Triaminic 1 teaspoon 3 times a day for the nasal congestion, which promoted the ear infection, to wean from the breastfeeding, as we mentioned, and to return to the clinic.

PROCEDURE NOTE

PREOPERATIVE DIAGNOSIS: Left peritonsillar abscess.

POSTOPERATIVE DIAGNOSIS: Left peritonsillar abscess.

ANESTHESIA: Local.

INDICATIONS: The patient is a 27-year-old male with evidence of a left peritonsillar abscess. He has had a sore throat for 3 weeks, which was initially treated with amoxicillin for 10 days. The sore throat resolved but then recurred after stopping the amoxicillin and has progressed to the point where the patient has had difficulty swallowing even his own secretions. He denies any shortness of breath, but reports that his voice is changed. He has had a low-grade fever with a maximum temperature of 100.5.

PHYSICAL EXAMINATION: The examination of the oropharynx and oral cavity reveals a marked swelling of the left peritonsillar area with deviation of the uvula to the right. He has bilateral tonsillar hypertrophy with erythema, but no exudate.

I recommended he undergo an incision and drainage of the left peritonsillar abscess immediately. The nature, course, and complications, including bleeding, infection, recurrence, and need for further treatment, were explained, and consent was obtained.

PROCEDURE: The oropharynx was sprayed with Cetacaine spray. The left peritonsillar area was then injected with a total of 2 mL of 1% lidocaine with 1:100,000 epinephrine solution. A #11 blade was used to incise the left peritonsillar area. Approximately 5 mL of tan, foul-smelling pus was drained, and culture was obtained. A hemostat was used to spread inside the incision to break up the loculations of the abscess cavity. The patient noted much relief of the pressure and pain in the left side of his throat after the procedure. He was monitored in the office for 20 minutes, and all bleeding was stopped prior to discharge from the office.

He was given a prescription for Augmentin 500 mg p.o. b.i.d. for 2 weeks. He was also given a prescription for Lortab 5 mg 1 p.o. q.4 h. p.r.n. pain. He is to follow up in my office in 1 week. He is to return to the office immediately or contact me if he develops any fever, bleeding, severe pain or swelling, difficulty breathing, or inability to take a satisfactory amount of liquids by mouth.

CLINIC NOTE

NOTE TO STUDENT: THIS NOTE USES A SECOND FORM OF THE "SOAP" FORMAT.

SUBJECTIVE: The patient is a 38-year-old female who is here for followup of pneumonia ×2 and possible infectious mononucleosis. The patient states that since her Floxin, she has developed a purulent sinus discharge and a cough. The patient is somewhat concerned about this and she feels upset because she has been treated for 2 months now. First, the patient was treated with amoxicillin and a course of erythromycin, and then later with Floxin. She denies shortness of breath, but does feel somewhat tired at this point.

OBJECTIVE: GENERAL: An alert female in no acute distress. VITAL SIGNS: Temperature 98.8 degrees Fahrenheit, blood pressure 100/60. HEAD, EARS, EYES, NOSE, AND THROAT EXAM: The right tympanic membrane is very distended, with a cloudy yellowish fluid behind it, and the canal is very red, inflamed, tender, and moderately swollen. The left tympanic membrane is clear. The throat is inflamed. There are no exudates. NECK EXAM: Tender retroauricular and anterior neck adenopathy. CHEST EXAM: Entirely clear. Initially there were some rhonchi heard in the left lower lobe, but these cleared with coughing. ABDOMEN: Soft and nontender. PELVIC: Deferred. EXTREMITIES: Without edema. NEUROLOGIC: Unremarkable.

ASSESSMENT: Acute right otitis media and externa.

PLAN:
1. Unasyn 1.5 g intramuscular.
2. Erythromycin 500 mg q.i.d. orally.
3. Percocet for pain as needed.
4. Return to the office or emergency room for worsening or for no improvement after 2 days.

EXERCISE TREADMILL TEST

This is a 40-year-old gentleman status post aortic valve replacement secondary to endocarditis who is undergoing exercise treadmill testing as part of an entrance to a cardiac rehabilitation program.

MEDICATIONS:

1. Metoprolol 50 mg b.i.d.
2. Lanoxin 0.25 mg daily.
3. Zoloft 50 mg daily.
4. Aspirin.

PROTOCOL: Standard Bruce protocol.

RESTING EKG: PR interval 0.16. QRS 0.06. Axis +90 degrees.

Interpretation: Sinus rhythm, rate of 76. Minor diffuse, nonspecific ST and T-wave abnormalities.

RESULTS: Patient exercised for 9 minutes, achieving a maximal heart rate of 140, which was 78% of his maximal predicted heart rate. Patient achieved 10 METS of exercise.

BLOOD PRESSURE: Initial resting blood pressure 118/78 and rose to a peak of 155/60 at peak exercise, then decreased to 138/75 five minutes in the recovery phase. Double product 21,700.

SYMPTOMS: Patient experienced leg fatigue while on the treadmill, but denied any chest tightness complaints.

REASON FOR STOPPING: Leg fatigue.

STRESS EKG: There were no ST or T-wave abnormalities suggestive of ischemia.

ARRHYTHMIAS: There were no PVCs, PACs, or supraventricular or ventricular tachycardia noted.

IMPRESSION:

1. Good exercise tolerance.
2. Negative for development of chest discomfort.
3. Electrocardiogram nondiagnostic, less than 85% of maximal predicted heart rate.
4. Normal blood pressure response.

APPENDIX D

Medical Transcription Projects Progress Sheet

STUDENT NAME:

Assignment	Date Completed	Grade
PROJECT 1 - OTORHINOLARYNGOLOGY		
Task 1-1A: True/False Exercise		
Task 1-1B: Combining Forms Exercise		
Task 1-1C: Medical Comprehension Exercise		
Task 1-2: Proofreading Exercises		
Cloze Exercise 1: Clinic Note_Report 6182		
Cloze Exercise 2: Clinic Note_Report 6103		
Transcription Exercise 1: Clinic Note_Report 6142		
Transcription Exercise 2: Clinic Note_Report 6119		
Transcription Exercise 3: Procedure Note_Report 6146		
Transcription Exercise 4: Operative Report_Report 6171		
Transcription Exercise 5: Letter_Report 6114		
SRT Exercise 1: Clinic Note_Report 13		
SRT Exercise 2: Clinic Note_Report 21		
SRT Exercise 3: MRI/MRA_Report 7		
SRT Exercise 4: Clinic Note_Report 7		
PROJECT 2 - OPHTHALMOLOGY		
Task 2-1A: Matching Exercise		
Task 2-1B: Multiple-Choice Exercise		
Task 2-1C: Spelling Choice Exercise		
Task 2-2: Proofreading Exercises		

Cloze Exercise 1: Clinic Note _Report 6		
Cloze Exercise 2: Clinic Note_Report 7		
Transcription Exercise 1: Clinic Note_Report 16		
Transcription Exercise 2: Clinic Note_Report 1		
Transcription Exercise 3: Clinic Note_Report 2		
Transcription Exercise 4: Operative Note_Report 1		
SRT Exercise 1: Operative Report _Report S-20		
SRT Exercise 2: Operative Report _Report 6		
PROJECT 3 - PULMONOLOGY		
Task 3-1A: Soundalike Term Review Exercise		
Task 3-1B: Fill in the Blanks Exercise		
Task 3-1C: Abbreviations Exercise		
Task 3-2: Proofreading Exercises		
Cloze Exercise 1: Chest X-ray_Report 3341		
Cloze Exercise 2: Clinic Note_Report 11		
Transcription Exercise 1: Clinic Note_Report 9001		
Transcription Exercise 2: Discharge Summary_Report 5		
Transcription Exercise 3: Clinic Note_Report 4		
Transcription Exercise 4: Clinic Note_Report 5		
Transcription Exercise 5: Clinic Note_Report 2		
SRT Exercise 1: Emergency Room Note_Report 9		
SRT Exercise 2: CT Scan of the Chest_Report 3213		
SRT Exercise 3: Discharge Summary_Report 2		
SRT Exercise 4: Discharge Summary_Report 3		
PROJECT 4 - CARDIOLOGY		
Task 4-1A: Medical Comprehension Exercise		
Task 4-1B: Combining Forms Exercise		
Task 4-1C: Fill in the Blanks Exercise		
Task 4-2: Proofreading Exercises		
Cloze Exercise 1: Progress Note_Report 7106		
Cloze Exercise 2: Exercise Treadmill Test _Report 7154		
Transcription Exercise 1: Admission History and Physical_Report 7124		
Transcription Exercise 2: 2-D Echocardiogram_Report 7119		
Transcription Exercise 3: 24-hour Holter Monitor_Report 7178		
Transcription Exercise 4: Adenosine Thallium Stress Test_Report 7167		
Transcription Exercise 5: Discharge Summary_Report 7196		

SRT Exercise 1: Progress Note_Report 7102		
SRT Exercise 2: History and Physical Examination_Report 7168		
SRT Exercise 3: Progress Note_Report 7120		
SRT Exercise 4: 2-D Echocardiogram_Report 7172		
PROJECT 5 - GASTROENTEROLOGY		
Task 5-1A: Fill in the Blanks Exercise		
Task 5-1B: Matching Exercise		
Task 5-1C: Multiple Choice Exercise		
Task 5-2: Proofreading Exercises		
Cloze Exercise 1: Operative Note_Report 5		
Cloze Exercise 2: Letter_Report 5118[2]		
Transcription Exercise 1: Progress Note_Report 5173[1]		
Transcription Exercise 2: Operative Note_Report 4		
Transcription Exercise 3: Endoscopy_Report 5132		
Transcription Exercise 4: Consultation, with Flexible Sigmoidoscopy_Report 5128		
Transcription Exercise 5: History and Physical, with EGD_Report 5161		
SRT Exercise 1: Operative Note_Report 2		
SRT Exercise 2: Discharge Summary_Report 5145		
SRT Exercise 3: Letter_Report 5126[2]		
SRT Exercise 4: Clinic Note_Report 4		
PROJECT 6 - OBSTETRICS and GYNECOLOGY		
Task 6-1A: True/False Exercise		
Task 6-1B: Medical Word Building Exercise		
Task 6-1C: Matching Exercise		
Task 6-2: Proofreading Exercises		
Cloze Exercise 1: Bilateral Mammograms_Report 3267		
Cloze Exercise 2: Clinic Note_Report 6		
Transcription Exercise 1: Clinic Note_Report 8		
Transcription Exercise 2: Operative Note_Report 3		
Transcription Exercise 3: Discharge Summary_Report 3		
Transcription Exercise 4: Operative Note_Report 13		
Transcription Exercise 5: Discharge Summary_Report 4		
SRT Exercise 1: Left Breast Sonogram_Report 3223		

SRT Exercise 2: Clinic Note_Report 4		
SRT Exercise 3: Clinic Note_Report 37		
SRT Exercise 4: Clinic Note_Report 63		
PROJECT 7 - UROLOGY		
Task 7-1A: Soundalike Term Review Exercise		
Task 7-1B: Fill in the Blanks Exercise		
Task 7-1C: Multiple Choice Exercise		
Task 7-2: Proofreading Exercises		
Cloze Exercise 1: Progress Note_Report 2130		
Cloze Exercise 2: Progress Note_Report 2183		
Transcription Exercise 1: History and Physical_Report 2133		
Transcription Exercise 2: Letter_Report 2174		
Transcription Exercise 3: Abdominal X-ray_Report 3143		
Transcription Exercise 4: Excretory Urogram_Report 3180		
Transcription Exercise 5: Clinic Note_Report 11		
SRT Exercise 1: History and Physical_Report 2118		
SRT Exercise 2: Letter_Report 2140		
SRT Exercise 3: Progress Note_Report 2138		
SRT Exercise 4: Progress Note_Report 2143		
PROJECT 8 - ORTHOPEDICS		
Task 8-1A: Matching Exercise		
Task 8-1B: Fill in the Blanks Exercise		
Task 8-1C: Matching Exercise		
Task 8-2: Proofreading Exercises		
Cloze Exercise 1: Lumbar MRI_Report 8		
Cloze Exercise 2: SOAP Note_Report 22		
Transcription Exercise 1: Consultation_Report 1		
Transcription Exercise 2: Clinic Note_Report 8		
Transcription Exercise 3: MRI_Report 10		
Transcription Exercise 4: SOAP Note_Report 7		
Transcription Exercise 5: Preoperative History and Physical_Report 13		
SRT Exercise 1: Bone Scan_Report 12		
SRT Exercise 2: Discharge Summary_Report 5		
SRT Exercise 3: Discharge Summary_Report 6		
SRT Exercise 4: Clinic Note_Report 7		

PROJECT 9 - DERMATOLOGY		
Task 9-1A: Fill in the Blanks Exercise		
Task 9-1B: Medical Word Building Exercise		
Task 9-1C: Multiple Choice Exercise		
Task 9-2: Proofreading Exercises		
Cloze Exercise 1: SOAP Note_Report 5		
Cloze Exercise 2: Clinic Note_Report 17		
Transcription Exercise 1: Operative Note_Report 14		
Transcription Exercise 2: Discharge Summary_Report 11		
Transcription Exercise 3: Procedure Note_Report 4		
Transcription Exercise 4: Discharge Summary_Report 2		
Transcription Exercise 5: History and Physical _Report 12		
SRT Exercise 1: SOAP Note_Report 4		
SRT Exercise 2: Discharge Summary_Report 10		

PROJECT 10 - NEUROLOGY		
Task 10-1A: Multiple Choice Exercise		
Task 10-1B: Medical Comprehension Exercise		
Task 10-1C: Matching Exercise		
Task 10-2: Proofreading Exercises		
Cloze Exercise 1: Clinic Note_Report 12		
Cloze Exercise 2: Clinic Note_Report 31		
Transcription Exercise 1: Brain Scan_Report 9		
Transcription Exercise 2: Letter_Report 11		
Transcription Exercise 3: Clinic Note_Report 9027		
Transcription Exercise 4: CT Scan of the Brain_Report 3102		
Transcription Exercise 5: Clinic Note_Report 9031		
SRT Exercise 1: Clinic Note_Report 9013		
SRT Exercise 2: X-Ray Report_Report 3133		

PROJECT 11 - ONCOLOGY		
Task 11-1A: Medical Comprehension Exercise		
Task 11-1B: Combining Forms Exercise		
Task 11-1C: Matching Exercise		
Task 11-2: Proofreading Exercises		
Cloze Exercise 1: Discharge Summary_Report 7		
Cloze Exercise 2: Chest X-ray and Isotope Bone Scan_Report 11		
Transcription Exercise 1: Discharge Summary_Report 4		
Transcription Exercise 2: Operative Note_Report 9		
Transcription Exercise 3: Letter_Report 15		
Transcription Exercise 4: Discharge Summary_Report 7		
Transcription Exercise 5: Abdominal Sonogram_Report 3385		
SRT Exercise 1: Clinic Note_Report 6		
SRT Exercise 2: Clinic Note_Report 9039		
SRT Exercise 3: Clinic Note_Report 6196		
SRT Exercise 4: Clinic Note_Report 9045		

PROJECT 12 - IMMUNOLOGY		
Task 12-1A: Matching Exercise		
Task 12-1B: Spelling Choice Exercise		
Task 12-1C: Medical Word Building Exercise		
Task 12-2: Proofreading Exercises		
Cloze Exercise 1: Clinic Note_Report 66		
Cloze Exercise 2: Clinic Note_Report 23		
Transcription Exercise 1: Discharge Summary _Report 8		
Transcription Exercise 2: Operative Note_Report 6		
Transcription Exercise 3: Clinic Note_Report 10		
Transcription Exercise 4: Clinic Note_Report 22		
Transcription Exercise 5: Thyroid Sonogram_Report 3363		
SRT Exercise 1: Clinic Note_Report 1		
SRT Exercise 2: Clinic Note_Report 30		

GLOSSARY

A

abdominal aorta The portion of the aorta that passes through the general area of the stomach in the body.

abdominal hysterectomy A hysterectomy that is performed through access from the abdomen.

abduction Movement of a limb away from the middle of the body.

aberration Visual distortions that cause the inability of light rays entering the eye to come together to a single focus point on the retina.

ABG (arterial blood gas) test A test in which a sample of blood is taken from an artery, usually at the wrist, that measures the levels of oxygen and carbon dioxide in the blood to determine how well a patient's lungs are working.

ablation A surgical treatment that removes or destroys the function of an organ or tissue.

abortus The number of pregnancy losses before the 20th week.

abscess A closed pocket containing pus.

absence seizure, *syn.* **petit mal seizure** A type of generalized seizure characterized by a brief loss of consciousness without associated motor symptoms.

accelerations An increase in the fetal heart rate.

access The site on the body where blood will be removed and returned during dialysis.

accessory muscles The muscles of the neck and chest not normally associated with breathing.

accessory organs The structures in the abdomen that are not part of the digestive tract but have a role in digestive activities necessary for the processing of food—specifically, the salivary glands, liver, gallbladder, and pancreas.

accommodation Ability of the eye to change its focus between distant objects and near objects.

acetabulum The socket in the hip bone that forms the ball-and-socket joint with the femur.

acetic acid A vinegar-like solution spray applied to the cervix during colposcopy to make abnormal tissues turn white.

acetowhite lesions Abnormal changes in the vagina and cervix that appear white after being sprayed with acetic acid.

Achilles tendonitis Inflammation of the Achilles tendon, which is the tendon that attaches the calf muscle to the back of the calcaneus, or heel bone.

acid-fast bacilli The physical property of certain bacteria that resist decolorization by acids during staining procedures, making them difficult to characterize using standard microbiological techniques.

ACL One of the four major ligaments located in the knee.

acne A chronic disorder of the hair follicles and sebaceous glands characterized by black heads, pimple outbreaks, cysts, infected abscesses, and sometimes scarring.

acoustic neurinoma A benign tumor that develops on the hearing and balance nerves of the ear, which can cause gradual hearing loss, tinnitus, and dizziness.

acquired hydrocephalus Hydrocephalus that can occur at any time after birth.

acquired immunodeficiency syndrome (AIDS) An often fatal disease of the immune system caused by the human immunodeficiency virus (HIV), which damages the immune system to the extent that opportunistic infections and cancers can attack the body.

active immunity The body's response and defense against pathogens it has encountered before.

Acuity In ophthalmology, a term that relates to sharpness, acuteness, or keenness of vision.

acute The sudden onset of symptoms or disease.

acute hepatitis A form of hepatitis that begins suddenly and has a limited course.

acute pancreatitis The sudden inflammation of the pancreas.

acute renal failure The sudden loss of the kidneys to excrete wastes.

acute respiratory distress syndrome (ARDS) A life-threatening condition in which inflammation of the lungs and accumulation of fluid in the alveoli leads to low blood oxygen levels.

adaptive immune system A system of highly specialized systemic cells that can recognize what belongs in the body and what does not, and remember specific pathogens in order to mount stronger attacks each time the pathogen is encountered.

adduction The movement of a limb toward the midline of the body.

adenocarcinoma Cancer that starts in epithelial tissue, such as the surface layer of skin, glands, and other tissue that lines the cavities and organs of the body.

adenoids Two clumps of lymphoid tissue located in the back of the nasal passages.

adenoma A benign or malignant tumor made up of glandular tissue.

adhesions Bands of fibrous scar tissue that form on organs.

adjuvant chemotherapy Chemotherapy given in addition to surgery or radiation therapy.

adnexa (of the uterus) Appendages or adjunct parts consisting of the fallopian tubes, ovaries, and the ligaments that hold them together.

adrenal gland A gland on top of each kidney that produces hormones which control metabolism, fluid balance, and blood pressure as well as androgens, estrogens, and progesterone.

adventitious sounds Abnormal breath sounds heard on lung examination.

afferent nerves Nerve fibers that carry sensory information from the peripheral nervous system to the central nervous system.

age-related macular degeneration (AMD) A disease that is caused by the malfunction of the photosensitive cells in the macula, causing distortion of images in the center of the visual field, darkened area in the center of an image, and diminished color a perception.

ala (plural *alae*) The flared cartilage on each side of the nostril.

alcoholic hepatitis An inflammation of the cells of the liver from alcohol abuse.

aldolase An enzyme tested to measure the amount of muscle damage in the body.

allergen A specific environmental antigen that initiates an allergic response.

allergy An abnormal reaction to a specific environmental antigen.

allogeneic bone marrow transplant A bone marrow transplant that uses marrow taken from another person and that is later infused back into the patient.

allograft A graft of bone or tissue between individuals of the same species. Allografts are usually obtained from cadaver.

alopecia Loss of hair. This can include all body hair besides scalp hair and can result from disease as well as certain type of cancer treatments.

alveoli Tiny sac-like air spaces in the lung where carbon dioxide and oxygen are exchanged.

amblyopia A condition in which the brain does not fully acknowledge the images seen by one eye, resulting in the abnormal development of visual pathways to the brain.

amenorrhea The absence or cessation of menstrual bleeding.

amniocentesis A test in which amniotic fluid is withdrawn from the uterus to test for genetic defects, infections, or lung immaturity in a fetus.

amniotic fluid A fluid that encases the fetus and provides a cushion for the fetus as the mother moves.

amputation The removal of an entire limb.

Amsler grid A grid of evenly spaced black horizontal and vertical lines on a sheet of white paper with a dot in the center, used to evaluate for macular problems.

amygdala The part of the limbic system that controls emotional reaction to a given situation.

amylase An enzyme produced by the pancreas that aids in digestion by breaking down starches.

analgesic A drug that relieves pain.

anastomosis The joining together of two healthy sections of tubular structures in the body after the diseased portion has been surgically removed.

androgen A male hormone.

anemia A deficiency in the red blood cells or concentrations of hemoglobin in body.

aneurysm An abnormal dilation of a blood vessel caused by a weakness in the vessel's wall.

angina, *syn.* **angina pectoris** Severe chest pain that results from an inadequate supply of oxygen and blood flow to the heart.

angiography A type of x-ray used to detect blockages in blood vessels using radioactive contrast.

angioma A benign tumor in the skin that is made up of blood or lymph vessels.

angioplasty, *syn.* **percutaneous transluminal coronary angioplasty (PTCA)** A procedure that opens narrowed arteries by use of a catheter with a balloon on its tip.

angiotensin II receptor blockers (ARBs) Drugs that block the action of the enzyme that causes blood vessels to narrow; similar to ACE inhibitors but without some of the side effects associated with ACE inhibitors.

angiotensin-converting enzyme (ACE) inhibitors A class of drugs that widen or dilate blood vessels to improve the amount of blood the heart pumps and lower blood pressure by inhibiting the formation of the enzymes angiotensin I and II, the chemicals that cause vessels to constrict.

ankle jerk The reflex tested by the tapping of the Achilles tendon of the foot with a short, sharp blow to the tendon with a tendon hammer.

ankylosing spondylitis A chronic inflammatory disease of the axial skeleton with involvement of peripheral joints and non-articular structures, mainly affecting the joints in the spine and sacroiliac joint in the pelvis.

annulus The tough outer ring of a spinal disk.

anosmia The absence of the sense of smell.

anoxia The total lack of oxygen supply.

antacid A medication that neutralizes stomach acids.

antalgic (gait) A limping-type gait.

anterior chamber The smaller front section of the eye filled with fluid that nourishes the internal structures of the eye and helps maintain its shape and pressure.

anterior communicating artery (AComA) A short artery that joins the two anterior cerebral arteries in the brain.

anterior cruciate ligament (ACL) The ligament located in the center of the knee that controls rotation and forward movement of the tibia (or shin bone).

anterior fontanel The area, sometimes called a *soft spot*, located toward the front and at the top of an infant's head, between the growing skull bones.

anterior horn The front third of the meniscus in the knee.

antibiotic A drug used to inhibit the growth of organisms that cause infection.

antibodies A type of protein produced by the immune system in response to foreign substances that may be a threat to the body.

anticardiolipin (aCL) An antiphospholipid antibody that causes damage to blood vessels and acts against proteins in the blood promoting clotting problems.

anticoagulant, *syn.* **blood thinner** A substance that hinders the clotting of blood.

antidiuretic hormone (ADH) A hormone that is released when the amount of water in the body decreases.

anti-double-stranded DNA A test that tags antibodies which bind to DNA.

antiemetic A drug that prevents or controls nausea and vomiting.

antifungal A drug used to treat fungal infections.

antigen A substance, such as chemicals, viruses, or bacteria, that causes the body's immune system to react by producing antibodies.

anti-La A specific type of autoantibody that helps to narrow down the diagnosis of a particular autoimmune disorder.

antineoplastic A drug that prevents, kills, or blocks the growth or spread of cancer cells.

antinuclear antibody (ANA) An antibody that reacts with a cell's nucleus, or command center.

antiphospholipid antibodies (APLs) Antibodies that cause damage to blood vessels and act against proteins in the blood to promote clotting problems.

antiretroviral drugs Medications that work to reduce the level of HIV in the blood, which, in turn, can dramatically slow the destruction of the immune system.

anti-Ro A specific type of autoantibody that helps to narrow down the diagnosis of a particular autoimmune disorder.

anti-Sm Dictated as *anti-Smith*, a specific type of autoantibody that helps to narrow down the diagnosis of a particular autoimmune disorder.

antrectomy The surgical removal of the lower part of the stomach.

antrum The lower portion of the stomach where grinding of food into smaller pieces takes place.

anus The opening at the end of the digestive tract through which stool leaves the body.

aorta The main trunk of the arterial system that begins in the left ventricle.

aortic valve The outgoing valve of the left ventricle.

apex The lowest superficial part of the heart, directed downward, forward, and to the left, and is overlapped by the left lung and pleura.

Apgar score The score of the Apgar test, which rates a newborn's physical condition immediately after birth.

aphakia The absence of the lens of the eye.

aphasia Difficulty with, or loss of use of language, in any of several ways, including reading, writing, or speaking, or the failure of understanding of the written, printed, or spoken word not related to intelligence but to specific lesions in the brain.

apheresis A procedure whereby whole blood is removed from the body and a desired component is retained, whereas the remainder of the blood is returned to the donor.

aphonia The complete loss of voice.

aplastic anemia A condition in which the bone marrow is unable to produce blood cells.

apnea Absence of breathing.

apoptosis The process of natural cell death that eliminates injured or genetically damaged cells.

appendicular skeleton The bones of the limbs as well as the shoulder and pelvic girdles of the skeleton.

appendix A small pouch of tissue that extends from the large intestine containing lymphoid tissue that scientists believe may be useful in fighting infection.

applanation tonometry A procedure that measures the pressure in the eye when evaluating for glaucoma.

aqueous humor Transparent fluid occupying the anterior chamber of the eye that functions to maintain adequate pressure in the eye.

arachnoid membrane The middle layer of membranes covering the brain and spinal cord.

Argon laser A device used to treat glaucoma (usually open angle) and diabetic retinopathy using a thermal beam.

arrector pili muscles Smooth muscle cells that surround hair follicles.

arrhythmia Any heart rhythm that falls outside the accepted norms with respect to rate or regularity.

arterial blood gas (ABG) A test performed to determine the amounts of oxygen and carbon dioxide dissolved in the blood, and to ascertain the acid base status of the blood.

arteries Larger vessels that carry oxygen-rich blood away from the heart. The exception is the pulmonary artery, which carries deoxygenated blood from the heart to the lungs.

arterioles Smaller branches of the arteries that distribute blood to body tissues.

arteriovenous Relating to both arteries and veins.

arteriovenous (AV) fistula An opening artificially created between an artery and vein to provide adequate blood flow for dialysis.

arteriovenous (AV) graft A synthetic tube used as an artificial vein connected to an artery to provide adequate blood flow for dialysis.

arteriovenous malformation (AVM) A collection of blood vessels with one or several abnormal communications between arteries and veins, which may cause hemorrhage or seizures.

arthralgia Pain in the joints.

arthritis Inflammation of a joint, usually accompanied by pain, swelling, and sometimes change in structure.

arthrocentesis, *syn.* **joint aspiration** The aspiration of fluid from a joint for examination in the laboratory.

arthroplasty, *syn.* **joint replacement** A reconstructive surgical procedure in which a diseased joint is replaced with long-lasting artificial parts to restore motion.

arthroscope An endoscopic instrument used to magnify and illustrate the structures inside a joint.

arthroscopy A minimally invasive diagnostic and treatment procedure used to visualize, diagnose, and treat problems inside a joint.

articular Referring to a joint (in RA, the disease affecting only the joints).

artificial skin graft A skin substitute derived from synthetic materials created in the laboratory used to help close wounds and aid in regeneration of a patient's native skin.

arytenoids Paired cartilages in the larynx that lie on top of the cricoid cartilage.

ascending colon The right-sided portion of the colon extending from the cecum to the hepatic flexure.

ascites An abnormal collection of fluid in the abdomen from cancer or other causes.

aspiration The removal of fluid or tissue from a specific area of the body.

assist control mode (A/C) A ventilator setting in which the patient sets his or her own breathing rate, but if the rate falls below a certain rate, the ventilator takes over.

asthma A disease in which the lung airways are inflamed and react with an oversensitivity of the lungs and airways to certain triggers.

astigmatic keratotomy (AK) A procedure to improve vision similar to RK, but using a curved pattern of incisions into the cornea rather than a radial pattern.

astigmatism Structural defects of the eye in which the light rays from a viewed object do not meet in a single focal point, resulting in blurred images being sent to the brain.

astrocytes Small, star-shaped cells.

astrocytoma A tumor within the substance of the brain or spinal cord made up of astrocytes.

asymptomatic Not having any symptoms of a disease.

asystole The complete absence of a heartbeat.

ataxia Uncontrolled gait; inability to control and coordinate muscle activity.

atelectasis Decreased or absent air in the entire or part of a lung, resulting in lung collapse.

atherectomy A procedure in which a high-speed drill on the tip of a catheter is used to shave plaque from blocked arterial walls.

atherosclerosis A buildup of fat-containing deposits called plaques on the walls of the coronary arteries, causing the arteries to become hardened and narrowed.

atopic dermatitis, *syn.* **eczema** A skin disorder that is characterized by itching, scaling, thickening of the skin, and is usually located on the face, elbows, knees, and arms.

atrial fibrillation A very fast, irregular heart rhythm that starts in the atria.

atrial flutter An arrhythmia in which the atrial rhythm is regular, but the rate is abnormally fast.

atrial septal defect (ASD) A hole in the atrium septum that separates the atria of the heart.

atrial tachycardia A rapid heart rate that starts in the atria (can be atrial flutter or atrial fibrillation).

atrioventricular (AV) node The electrical connection between the atria and ventricles where electrical impulses are delayed for a fraction of a second to allow the ventricles to fill completely with blood.

Atrium (plural *atria*) The name given to each of the two upper chambers of the heart that collect blood returning from the rest of the body and pass it to the ventricles.

atrophy A wasting of the tissues of a body part.

atypical Not usual or abnormal.

audiologist A healthcare professional trained to identify and measure hearing impairments and related disorders using a variety of tests and procedures.

audiology The diagnosis of disease through the evaluation of hearing loss.

aura A subjective warning sign that occurs immediately before the onset of a seizure.

auscultation The process of listening to heart sounds through a stethoscope.

autoantibodies Abnormal antibodies produced against the body's own tissues.

autograft A graft of bone or skin obtained from the patient for transplantation elsewhere on the patient.

autoimmunity An abnormal condition in which the immune system confuses normal body tissue (self) and attacks the tissues of the body, causing pain and loss of function.

autologous bone marrow transplant A bone marrow transplant that uses marrow taken directly from the donor patient.

autosomal dominant polycystic kidney disease (ADPKD) An inherited form of polycystic kidney disease (PKD).

avascular A term meaning without blood or lymphatic vessels.

avascular necrosis (AVN), *syn.* **osteonecrosis** The death of bone tissue due to a permanent loss of blood supply.

avulsion Tearing away. A nerve can be avulsed by an injury, as can part of a bone.

axial skeleton The skeleton that includes the bones of the skull, vertebral column, and chest.

axilla Another name for the armpit.

B

B cells A type of lymphocyte that matures in the bone marrow and makes antibodies that destroy bacteria, viruses, and other foreign substances that enter the body.

Babinski test A type of reflex test that involves gently stroking the sole of the foot to assess proper development of the spine and cerebral cortex.

bacteremia The presence of bacteria in the blood.

bacterial endocarditis An infection leading to deformity and/or destruction of the inner layer of the heart.

bacterial meningitis An infection by bacteria causing inflammation of the meninges.

bacterial pneumonia A pneumonia caused by bacteria.

bacteruria The presence of bacteria in the urine.

barrel chest A chest expanded in the shape of a barrel, a condition often seen in COPD patients due to chronic hyperinflation of the lungs.

Barrett esophagus A precancerous condition of the lower esophagus as a result of chronic damage to the lining of the esophagus, increasing the risk of cancer.

Bartholin glands Glands that keep the vaginal mucosa moist and provide a lubricant for the vagina during sexual intercourse.

basal cell carcinoma The most common form of skin cancer beginning in the basal cells of the epidermis.

basal cells Living cells found in the basal layer of the skin.

basal ganglia Islands of nerve cell clusters embedded in the white matter of the brain.

Becker muscular dystrophy (BMD) A common form of muscular dystrophy in children and a milder form of the disease.

Bell palsy An idiopathic attack on the facial nerve, causing sudden weakness or paralysis of the muscles on one side of the face.

benign A term describing a tumor that is noncancerous or harmless.

benign paroxysmal positional vertigo (BPPV), *syn.* **vertigo** A sensation of dizziness as a result of a disorder or a blockage in the structures of the inner ear.

benign prostatic hyperplasia, *syn.* **benign prostatic hypertrophy (BPH)** An enlargement of the prostate caused by disease or inflammation. It is not cancer, but its symptoms are often similar to those of prostate cancer.

beta-blockers A class of drugs that slow the heart rate and reduce the force of the heartbeat by dilating the arteries.

beta hCG A hormone that is detected in a urine test to indicate pregnancy.

bicarbonate (HCO₃) A buffer in the blood that keeps the pH within a normal range.

bigeminy A repeating pattern of one normal contraction of the heart followed by one premature contraction.

bilateral salpingo-oophorectomies (BSO) The surgical removal of both fallopian tubes and ovaries.

bile A yellow-brown fluid produced by the liver that assists in the digestion and absorption of fats and is responsible for the elimination of waste products from the body.

biliary tract A series of ducts which, along with the gallbladder, convey and store bile.

bilirubin A chemical formed from the degradation of hemoglobin in the blood, which is processed by the liver and then secreted into the bile.

Billroth I procedure, *syn.* **gastroduodenostomy** A procedure that involves the surgical removal of the lower part of the stomach and attaching the remaining portion to the duodenum.

Billroth II procedure, *syn.* **gastrojejunostomy** A procedure that involves surgically removing the lower part of the stomach and attaching the remaining portion to the jejunum.

biopsy The removal of cells or tissues for examination by a pathologist, who studies the tissue under a microscope to help a health provider to diagnose a medical disease or condition.

BI-RADS A system developed by radiologists to report mammogram results using a common language.

bisphosphonates A family of drugs developed to inhibit bone breakdown.

bladder distention A procedure whereby the bladder is inflated with gas or liquid.

bladder instillation A procedure whereby the bladder is inflated with the chemical compound DMSO to reduce inflammation and pain.

bladder neck The opening from the trigone, which contains the opening into the urethra.

bladder reconstruction A surgical procedure in which a section of bowel is made into a balloon-shaped sac and connected to the top of the urethra so that urine can be stored and drained from the body normally.

bleb A blister-like sac filled with blood.

blepharitis Inflammation of the eyelids, a common problem that tends to be recurrent in nature.

blind spot The area of the optic disc where the optic nerve fibers exit the eye and where there are no light-sensitive cells.

blister A fluid-filled bump on the skin.

blood-brain barrier A system of central nervous system (CNS) capillaries that prevent many substances from entering the brain and/or spinal cord, acting as a selective filter to limit harmful substances into the brain.

blood pressure The force of blood exerted on the inside walls of blood vessels.

blood urea nitrogen (BUN) A substance produced from the breakdown of food protein and a measure of the kidneys' ability to excrete urea.

blood vessels A network of interconnecting arterial, arterioles, capillaries, venules, and veins that provides the pathway in which blood is transported between the heart and body cells.

body The large central part of the stomach. It may also refer to the upper part of the uterus that lies below the entrance to the fallopian tubes or the middle third of the meniscus of the knee.

boil A warm, painful, pus-filled pocket of infection below the skin's surface.

bolus A single dose of drug usually injected into a blood vessel over a short period of time.

bone Hard connective tissue that makes up the skeleton.

bone densitometry A procedure that uses x-rays to measure the bone mass, or weight, of the skeleton.

bone flap A portion of the skull that is temporarily removed during a surgical procedure and replaced when the procedure is completed.

bone grafting A procedure in which bone tissue with the blood vessels intact from elsewhere in the body is attached to damaged bone tissue and blood vessels in order to serve as an infrastructure from which the body forms new bone.

bone marrow The soft spongy substance found inside bones that produces blood cells.

bone marrow biopsy A procedure in which a needle is inserted into a bone to take out a sample of bone marrow.

bone marrow transplant (BMT) A procedure in which marrow is taken from the bones of a patient before chemotherapy treatment and then put back into the patient later to replace the marrow that was destroyed by chemotherapy.

bone scan, *syn.* **radionuclide scan** A picture of all the bones in the body to detect abnormal processes involving the bone.

Bowman capsule Another name for *glomerular capsule.*

brachytherapy Internal radiation treatment given by placing radioactive material directly into the tumor or close to it.

bradycardia, *syn.* **bradyarrhythmia** A heart rate that is abnormally slow, commonly defined as under 60 beats per minute.

bradykinesia Slowness of body movement.

brain The part of the nervous system that is enclosed in the skull and connected to the spinal cord and includes all the body's higher nervous centers.

brainstem The lower extension of the brain that controls levels of consciousness and automatically regulates critical vital functions such as heartbeat and respirations.

brain tumor A mass of abnormal cells growing in the brain.

breast cancer A cancerous tumor of breast tissue.

breech presentation The baby's position in the uterus in which the baby is buttocks or feet first as opposed to head first.

bronchi (singular *bronchus*) The two main air passages that enter the right and left lung, respectively.

bronchiectasis The dilation of the large airways with the accumulation of secretions and chronic infection.

bronchioles The finer subdivisions of the branched bronchial tree.

bronchiolitis Inflammation of the bronchioles, usually caused by a viral infection.

Bronchitis An inflammation of the bronchi that causes increased production of mucus and other changes.

bronchoalveolar lavage (BAL) The process of washing the lining of the bronchi or bronchioles to obtain cells for culture to diagnose diseases.

bronchodilator A drug that relaxes the smooth muscles of the airways and relieves constriction of the bronchi.

bronchogenic carcinoma, *syn.* **lung cancer** A cancer of the bronchi of the airway.

bronchopneumonia An infection of the smaller bronchial tubes of the lungs.

bronchopulmonary Pertaining to the lungs and air passages.

bronchoscope A thin, tube-like instrument used to examine the inside of the trachea, bronchi (air passages that lead to the lungs), and lungs.

bronchoscopy The insertion of a flexible, lighted tube through the mouth and into the lungs allowing the physician to examine and take a biopsy of the lungs and bronchi (breathing tubes).

bronchus (plural *bronchi*) A large airway that leads from the trachea to either lung.

Bruce protocol The standardized treadmill stress test used for diagnosing and evaluating heart and lung diseases.

bruit An abnormal sound made by blood rushing past an obstruction in an artery.

B-type natriuretic peptide (BNP) A hormone originating in the heart that is released into the bloodstream in high levels when the heart is overworked over a long period of time (such as with heart failure).

bulb The onion-shaped structure at the end of the root of hair.

bulbourethral glands Pea-sized structures that produce a clear fluid that empties directly into the urethra to lubricate the urethra and neutralize any acidity that may be present from residual urine.

bulla (plural *bullae*) A large fluid-filled, honey colored blister.

bundle branch block An arrhythmia in which the electrical impulses of the heart are unable to travel down the right or left bundle of His.

bundle branches (right and left) Pathways that branch off the bundle of His that help carry the electrical signals of cardiac conduction to the ventricles.

bundle of His Specialized nerve fibers that help carry the electrical signals of cardiac conduction to the ventricles.

burn An injury to the skin caused by heat, electricity, chemicals, or radiation.

bursa A sac filled with fluid located between a bone and a tendon or muscle.

bursitis Repeated small stresses and overuse that cause the bursa to swell and become irritated.

C

cadaveric transplant A transplantation procedure in which the donated kidney comes from a dead person.

calcaneus The heel bone of the foot.

calcitriol An active form of vitamin D that helps increase the absorption of calcium and phosphorus from the small intestine.

calcium channel blockers A class of drugs that inhibit the movement of calcium ions into the muscle cells of the heart and arteries, resulting in a decrease in the force of the heart's pumping action and relaxing of muscle cells in the walls of the arteries, which helps them to open and to reduce blood pressure.

calyx (plural *calyces*) Funnel-shaped extension of the renal pelvis.

cancer A general term for a large group of diseases in which there is uncontrolled growth and spread of abnormal cells.

Candida Thin-walled, small yeasts that cause candidiasis.

candidiasis An infection caused by the *Candida* species of fungi.

capillaries Tiny thin-walled vessels that allow oxygen and nutrients to pass from blood to tissues.

carbuncles Clusters of abscesses that are connected to each other under the skin.

carcinogen A substance that causes cancer.

carcinoma A malignant tumor that begins in the lining layer (epithelial cells) of organs.

carcinoma in situ A cancer that has not spread to other areas of the body or nearby organs.

cardia The top portion of the stomach.

cardiac arrest A condition that occurs when the heart suddenly stops pumping effectively and begins to flutter wildly, failing to pump blood to the vital organs of the body.

cardiac catheterization A diagnostic procedure using a catheter threaded into the heart chambers that identifies possible problems with the heart or its arteries.

cardiac conduction The name given to the electrical conduction system that controls the heart rate.

cardiac cycle The sequence of events of one heartbeat.

cardiac ischemia The name for lack of blood flow and oxygen to the heart muscle.

cardiac muscle Muscle that is found only in the heart.

cardiac stress test, *syn.* **treadmill stress test** An exercise test that evaluates the heart for problems which appear when the heart is working hard.

cardiac tamponade Compression of the heart caused by blood or fluid accumulation in the space between the myocardium (the muscle of the heart) and the pericardium (the outer covering sac of the heart).

cardiology The medical specialty dealing with the diagnosis and treatment of diseases and disorders of the heart.

cardiomyopathy Progressive impairment of the structure and function of the myocardium.

cardiopulmonary A term relating to the heart and lungs.

cardiothoracic A term describing the relationship between the heart and thoracic cavity.

cardiovascular The circulatory system consisting of the heart and the blood vessels which carries nutrients and oxygen to the tissues of the body and removes carbon dioxide and other wastes from them.

cardioversion A medical procedure by which an abnormally fast heart rate or cardiac arrhythmia is converted to a normal rhythm by the use of electrical current or drugs.

carotid artery The large artery on either side of the neck which supplies most of the cerebral hemisphere.

carpals The eight small bones of the wrist that articulate with the distal ends of the ulna and radius and with the proximal ends of the metacarpals.

carpal tunnel syndrome A condition where the median nerve is cut off at the wrist because of compression of the nerve at the carpal ligament.

cartilage A smooth material that covers bone ends of a joint to cushion the bone and allow the joint to move easily without pain.

cartilaginous joints Joints that can only move slightly.

cataract Gradual clouding of the crystalline lens of the eye resulting in reduced vision or eventual blindness, correctable by cataract surgery.

catheter A small, thin, flexible tube.

cauda equina A bundle of nerves that extend beyond the end of the spinal cord.

cavernous hemangioma A raised red or purple mark in the skin, made up of enlarged blood vessels.

cecum The pouch at the beginning of the large intestine.

cell The structural and functional unit of which all living things are made.

cellulitis An acute bacterial infection of the skin and underlying tissues.

central nervous system (CNS) The division of the nervous system consisting of the brain and spinal cord.

cerebellum The lower part of the brain that is beneath the posterior portion of the cerebrum and regulates unconscious coordination of movement.

cerebral aneurysm A sac-like outpouching that can occur in the large arteries at the base of the brain.

cerebral angiogram A test used to detect an obstruction in a blood vessel or in the brain, head, or neck.

cerebral cortex A layer of millions of neurons and glia on the surface of the brain that carry out the many functions of the cerebrum.

cerebrospinal fluid (CSF) A clear fluid that flows in the cavities and around the surface of the brain as well as the spinal cord.

cerebrum The uppermost and largest part of the brain.

cerumen Ear wax.

cervical cancer A cancer that develops in the lining of the cervix.

cervical dysplasia The development of abnormal cells in the lining of the cervix.

cervical intraepithelial neoplasia (CIN) An alternative name for cervical dysplasia and a method to categorize the abnormal changes observed in cervical tissue.

cervical lymph nodes Lymph nodes in the neck.

cervical spine Upper spine, neck. Made up of seven vertebrae.

cervicitis An irritation of the cervix by a number of different organisms. Cervicitis is generally classified as either acute or chronic.

cervix The lower, narrow part of the uterus located between the bladder and the rectum. It forms a canal that opens into the vagina, which leads to the outside of the body.

cesarean section A method of delivery of a newborn through a surgical incision in the abdomen and front wall of the uterus.

chambers The compartments of the heart through which blood flows.

chemotherapy A treatment that involves anticancer drugs administered either intravenously or orally to kill cancer cells.

Cheyne-Stokes respirations A respiratory pattern that describes alternating periods of apnea and deep, rapid breathing.

chlamydia The most common type of sexually transmitted disease in the United States, named after the bacterium that causes the infection.

chlamydial infection A very common sexually transmitted disease or urinary tract infection caused by a bacteria like organism in the urethra and reproductive system.

cholangiopancreatography The portion of an ERCP procedure where x-rays are taken to document abnormalities in the bile ducts, gallbladder, or pancreas.

cholecystectomy The surgical removal of the gallbladder.

cholecystitis A sudden inflammation of the gallbladder.

choledocholithiasis A condition in which gallstones form inside the common bile duct.

cholelithiasis A condition in which gallstones form inside the gallbladder.

cholesteatoma Accumulation of dead cells in the middle ear, caused by repeated middle ear infections.

chondromalacia Abnormal softening or degeneration of cartilage.

chondrosarcoma A large, slow-growing malignant tumor that usually develops in the cartilage around the long bones of the body.

chordee A downward curve of the shaft of the penis.

choroid membrane Dark, vascular, thin, skin-like tissue situated between the sclera and the retina forming the middle coat of the eye. The choroid membrane nourishes the outer portions of the retina and absorbs excess light.

choroid plexus The vascular complex that lies along the floor of the lateral ventricles where CSF is produced.

chromosome Part of a cell that contains genetic information.

chronic Persisting over a long period of time.

chronic kidney failure A long-term condition in which the kidneys gradually and progressively lose their ability to function.

chronic obstructive pulmonary disease (COPD) A collective term for a group of respiratory tract diseases that are characterized by airflow limitation.

chronic pancreatitis A slow, ongoing inflammation of the pancreas that occurs when digestive enzymes attack and destroy the pancreas and nearby tissues over time, causing scarring and pain.

chronic sinusitis A condition in which the nasal sinuses become inflamed, causing improper drainage.

chyme A mushy liquid to which food is converted by the stomach.

cilia Tiny hairs within the cells of the bronchial-lining tissue.

ciliary body A thin, transparent capsule of muscular tissue containing the lens.

circulatory system A transportation system of blood vessels that circulates blood and other fluids throughout the body, delivers nutrients and other essential materials to cells, and removes waste products from the body.

circumduction A circular movement of a body part.

circumflex artery A branch of the left coronary artery in the heart situated along the left atrium on the outside of the heart wall.

cirrhosis A condition in which normal cells of the liver are damaged and replaced by scar tissue.

clavicle The bone that runs along the front of the shoulder to the breast bone (the collarbone).

clean catch The collection of a midstream sample of urine in a sterile container.

clear cell carcinoma A type of cancer that can originate in the uterus or the ovary.

climacteric, *syn.* **menopause** The transition period of time before menopause, marked by a decreased production of estrogen and progesterone, irregular menstrual periods, and transitory psychological changes.

clinical trial A planned scientific study of the effects of a diagnostic test or treatment on selected patients, usually with respect to safety, efficacy, and/or quality of life.

clitoris A small mass of erectile tissue in females that responds to sexual stimulation.

closed reduction Reduction by manipulation of bone without incising the skin and muscle over the site of the fracture.

clue cells Vaginal cells that appear fuzzy under a microscope when coated with bacteria, indicating infection.

coarctation A constriction, narrowing or compression.

cobblestone A lumpy appearance of mucosa similar to a cobblestone pathway.

coccyx The small bone at the end of the spinal column, formed by the fusion of four rudimentary vertebrae. The "tail bone."

cochlea A snail-shaped structure in the inner ear that contains the organ of hearing.

coil embolization A procedure whereby tiny platinum coils are placed directly into an aneurysm to block blood flow and prevent rupture.

cold knife cone biopsy A procedure in which a section of abnormal tissue along with normal-appearing tissue is removed from the cervix with a surgical scalpel and examined under a microscope.

colectomy The surgical removal of all or part of the colon.

collagen A major protein found in connective tissue, cartilage, and bone.

collateral vessels Preexisting blood vessels that help restore blood flow by bypassing areas of narrowing in other blood vessels.

colon The part of the large intestine that extends from the small intestine to the rectum.

colonoscope A flexible, elongated endoscope used to view the inside of the entire colon and rectum.

colonoscopy A procedure to look at the rectum and the colon by means of a lighted, flexible tube.

colorectal cancer A term used to refer to cancer that originates in the colon or rectum.

colostomy A surgical procedure by which an opening is created between the colon and the outside of the abdomen in order to eliminate stool into a collection bag.

colostrum A substance produced by the mammary glands that contains milk fat and immunoglobulins.

colposcope A lighted instrument used to identify and evaluate abnormal areas in the vagina and cervix.

colposcopy A procedure that uses a colposcope to view and evaluate abnormal areas in the vagina and cervix.

comminuted fracture A fracture in which bone is broken, splintered, or crushed into a number of pieces.

common bile duct The duct that carries bile from the liver and gallbladder into the duodenum.

communicating hydrocephalus A type of hydrocephalus that results from an actual problem with the actual production of CSF or absorption of CSF.

compact bone Tightly packed, hard material that makes up the outside surface of bones.

compensated heart failure A stage of congestive heart failure (CHF), a condition in which the patient's CHF becomes asymptomatic due to improved blood flow through the heart.

complement A collective term for a system of serum proteins designed to destroy foreign cells and help remove foreign materials.

complex partial seizures A type of partial seizure in which consciousness is altered during the seizure event.

compound fracture A fracture in which the bone is sticking through the skin.

computed tomography scan, *syn.* **CT scan** A diagnostic imaging procedure that uses a combination of x-rays and computer technology to produce cross-sectional images (often called *slices*), both horizontally and vertically, of the body that show detailed images of the body, including the bones, muscles, fat, and organs.

conchae (singular *concha*), *syn.* **nasal turbinates** The bony structures that form the posterior walls of the nasal passages.

concussion A disruption, usually temporary, of neurological function resulting from a blow or violent shaking.

conduction system A term that refers to the system of electrical signaling that instructs the muscle cells of the atria and ventricles to contract in near synchrony.

conduction velocity The speed of the response of motor or sensory nerve impulses during nerve conduction studies.

conductive keratoplasty (CK) A procedure to improve vision that shrinks the collagen in the cornea by using heat from low-level radiofrequency waves.

condyloma acuminata, *syn.* **genital warts** Warts that appear on or around the genitals.

cone biopsy, *syn.* **conization** A procedure in which a cone-shaped piece of abnormal tissue in the cervix is removed and examined under a microscope.

cones Cells in the photoreceptor layer that are responsible for fine color vision.

congenital Present at birth.

congenital hydrocephalus Hydrocephalus that is present at birth.

congestion Buildup of fluid in an organ or tissue.

congestive heart failure A condition that occurs when the heart's weak pumping action causes a buildup of fluid in the lungs and other body tissues.

conjunctiva (plural *conjunctivae*) Mucous membrane lining the inner surface of the eyelids and covering the front part of the sclera (white part of eye), responsible for keeping the eye moist.

conjunctivitis An infection of the conjunctival layer of the eye.

connective tissue Tissue that connects, supports, binds, or separates other tissues or organs.

contact dermatitis A rash or an inflammation of the skin caused by contact with various substances.

contusion Another name for a bruise.

convulsive (seizure) Relating to a type of seizure in which the body stiffens briefly, and then begins jerking movements.

cor Another term for "heart."

core biopsy The small piece of bone marrow obtained for microscopic examination.

core decompression A surgical procedure used to increase blood flow to bone in patients with avascular necrosis (AVN).

cornea The clear layer located at the front and center of the eye.

corneal topography A test that uses a computer to analyze the curvature of the cornea.

corneal transplant (penetrating keratoplasty) Surgical operation of grafting a replacement cornea onto an eye.

coronal suture The immobile joint that unites the frontal bone and two parietal bones of the skull.

coronary Relating to the heart, or to one of the two arteries that originate in the aorta and supply blood directly to heart tissue.

coronary angiography The part of the cardiac catheterization procedure in which a dye is inserted through the catheter to enable the viewing of images of the blood vessels as the heart pumps.

coronary arteries The network of blood vessels that supply oxygen-rich and nutrient-rich blood directly to the heart's muscle tissue.

coronary artery bypass graft (CABG) A surgical procedure in which a section of vein or artery from another part of the body is used to bypass a blockage in a coronary artery so that blood flow is not hindered.

coronary artery disease (CAD) The narrowing of the coronary arteries sufficiently to prevent adequate blood supply to the heart muscle; also called *cardiac ischemia*.

coronary thrombosis Damage to the heart muscle caused by a thrombus, or blood clot, blocking a coronary artery.

corpectomy Removal of the body of a vertebra. The body is the solid bony mass, almost circular in appearance, which forms the front part of each vertebra.

corpus callosum The fibrous band connecting the left and right hemispheres of the brain.

corpus luteum A temporary endocrine gland formed from an ovarian follicle that has released an ovum, which secretes progesterone during the second half of the menstrual cycle.

cortex The external layer of gray matter covering the hemispheres of the cerebrum and cerebellum.

corticosteroid Any of a number of steroid substances obtained from the cortex of the adrenal glands. They are sometimes used as an anti cancer treatment or to reduce persistent nausea.

costal cartilage The cartilage that occupies the spaces between the ribs and connects the ends of the ribs to the sternum.

Cowper glands Another name for the *bulbourethral glands*.

cranial bones The top part of the skull that encloses the brain.

cranial nerves Nerves that exit from the brain, which connect the brain with the eyes, ears, nose, and throat and with various parts of the head, neck, and trunk.

craniectomy Surgical removal of a portion of the skull.

craniopharyngioma A congenital tumor arising from the embryonic duct between the brain and pharynx.

cranioplasty The operative repair of a defect of the skull.

craniosynostosis Premature closure of cranial sutures, limiting or distorting the growth of the skull.

craniotomy Surgical opening of the skull, usually by creating a flap of bone.

C-reactive protein A substance in the blood that is secreted when inflammation in the artery walls occurs.

creatine kinase (CK), *syn.* **creatine phosphokinase (CPK)** A cardiac enzyme found in the heart that plays a major role in the production of energy in the body.

creatinine A waste product from meat protein and from normal wear and tear on the body.

creatinine clearance A test used to help evaluate the rate and efficiency of kidney filtration by the glomeruli.

crepitation A grating or crackling sound or sensation, as that produced by the fractured ends of a bone moving against each other.

Crohn disease A condition causing open sores affecting all layers lining the entire wall of the large and/or small intestine.

crossmatching antigen test A test that is performed to define how a kidney transplant recipient may respond to particular cells or proteins of the kidney donor.

cryoablation A procedure in which extreme cold is used to destroy cancerous tissue.

cryomyolysis A procedure in which liquid nitrogen is used to freeze and destroy a uterine fibroid.

cryopreservation The process of freezing an embryo prior to IVF transfer.

cryoprobe The instrument used to apply extreme cold to tissue.

cryosurgery The use of liquid nitrogen to destroy visible skin lesions. Commonly used for actinic keratoses, verruca vulgaris, and molluscum contagiosum.

crystalline lens A clear, flexible structure that allows for fine focusing of light as it passes through the eye.

C-section Another term for *cesarean section*.

CT myelogram A myelogram used in conjunction with a CT scan to examine the spinal cord and subarachnoid space.

culture A material or specimen obtained from the body and incubated with a nutrient medium to isolate organisms and determine the cause of an illness or infection.

curet (also spelled curette) A spoon-shaped instrument with a cutting edge and handle used to remove tissue in the body.

curettage The procedure or removal of a new growth or irregular tissue with a curette.

cutaneous The term that describes something relating to the skin.

cutaneous candidiasis An infection of the skin with *Candida*.

cyanosis Bluish color of the skin due to insufficient oxygen in the blood.

cyclooxygenase-2 (COX-2) inhibitors A class of NSAIDs that blocks the enzyme that causes pain and swelling of joints.

cyst A deep lesion that is filled with pus or other contents.

cystic duct The duct that joins the common bile duct to the gallbladder.

cystic fibrosis (CF) An inherited (genetic) condition affecting the cells that produce mucus, sweat, saliva, and digestive juices.

cysteine An organic building block that helps make up muscles, nerves, and other parts of the body.

cystitis An inflammation of the bladder caused by bacteria, chemotherapy or radiation treatments.

cystocele A condition that occurs when the wall between the bladder and the vagina weakens, causing the bladder to drop or sag into the vagina.

cystometer An instrument that is used to study the pressure and filling capacity of the bladder.

cystometrogram (CMG) A urodynamic study that measures the function and stability of the bladder.

Cystoscopy A procedure that examines structures of the urinary system.

cystoscopy, *syn.* **cystourethroscopy** An examination in which a scope, a flexible tube and viewing device, is inserted through the urethra to examine the bladder and urinary tract for structural abnormalities or obstructions, such as tumors or stones.

Cytokines Chemical messengers used by the cells of the immune system to communicate with one another to coordinate an appropriate immune response.

cytology The branch of science that deals with the structure and function of cells. It also refers to tests used to diagnose cancer and other diseases by examination of cells under the microscope.

cytomegalovirus (CMV) A virus that occurs in healthy individuals without causing symptoms, but in immunocompromised individuals, can cause pneumonia and other serious illnesses.

cytotoxic Toxic to cells; cell killing.

D

debridement The process of removing dead tissue to expose and cleanse the area.

debulking A procedure that removes a significant part or most of a tumor in cases where it is not possible to remove all of it. This may make subsequent radiotherapy or chemotherapy easier and more effective.

decannulation The removal of the breathing tube.

decelerations Decreases in the fetal heart rate.

decibel Unit that measures the intensity or loudness of sound.

decompensated heart failure A stage of congestive heart failure in which the myocardium of the heart becomes flabby and loses its ability to contract.

deep brain stimulation (DBS) A procedure that involves implanting a device to deliver mild electrical stimulation to block the brain signals that cause tremors in patients with Parkinson disease.

deep tendon reflexes (DTRs) A test of the deep tendons that can indicate pressure on or injury to the spinal cord.

deep venous thrombosis (DVT) Blood clots in leg veins.

defecation The discharge of solid waste from the body.

defibrillation Used to treat arrhythmia; a process of delivering a therapeutic dose of electrical energy to the affected heart with a device called a defibrillator that depolarizes a critical mass of the heart muscle, terminating the arrhythmia and allowing the heart to resume a normal sinus rhythm naturally.

degenerative disk disease Gradual or rapid deterioration of the chemical composition and physical properties of the disk space.

demyelination A gradual destruction of the myelin that surrounds and protects neurons.

depression A downward movement.

dermatitis A number of skin conditions characterized by inflammation of the skin.

dermatofibroma Small, red or brown bumps in the skin.

dermatomes Specific regions of the body which are supplied by the sensory nerve fibers of a single nerve root.

dermatophytes Microscopic organisms that live on keratin and cause a fungal infection in the skin.

dermis The middle layer of skin, which is made up of blood vessels, lymph vessels, hair follicles, and sweat glands.

dermoid cyst A benign tumor made up of hairs, sweat glands, and sebaceous glands.

descending colon The left-sided portion of the colon extending from the splenic flexure to the beginning of the sigmoid colon.

desiccation The application of an electrical current to an incision to control bleeding and kill remaining cancer cells.

desquamation The process of shedding dead skin cells from the epidermis and replenishing them from the deeper layers of the dermis.

detrusor muscle The outermost layer of muscle of the bladder.

diabetic retinopathy A degenerative eye disease in which diabetes causes damage to the blood vessels that nourish the retina.

diagonal branches (D_1, D_2) Lesser coronary vessels that branch off the left coronary artery.

dialysis A medical procedure that removes waste and additional fluid from the blood after the kidneys have stopped functioning.

diaphoresis An abnormal increase in the amount of sweat.

diaphragm The muscle that separates the thoracic cavity from the abdominal cavity that contracts and relaxes during breathing.

diaphysis The tubular shaft of a long bone.

diastole Normal period of relaxation and dilation of the heart chambers.

diastolic pressure The bottom number in a blood pressure reading that represents the minimum blood pressure as the heart relaxes following a contraction.

diffusing capacity for carbon monoxide (DLCO) The amount of carbon monoxide exhaled compared to the amount inhaled.

diffusion A process whereby oxygen passes from the blood to the tissue fluid and carbon dioxide moves from the tissue fluid to the blood to be brought back to the lungs and to be exhaled.

digestion The process by which food and liquid are broken down into smaller parts and converted into forms of energy the body can use to maintain life and health.

digestive disorders Diseases and medical problems affecting the gastrointestinal system.

dilatation The condition of being abnormally dilated or enlarged.

dilated cardiomyopathy A disease of the heart which causes weakening of the heart muscle and causes left ventricular dilation leading to increased diastolic pressure and volume.

dilation Another word for *enlargement*. It also refers to the opening of the cervix during labor.

dilation and curettage (also called **D&C**) A minor operation in which the cervix is dilated (expanded) so that the cervical canal and uterine lining can be scraped with a curette (spoon shaped instrument).

diopter Unit of measure of the refractive power of an optical lens (equal to the power of a lens with a focal distance of one meter). A negative diopter value (such as -3D) signifies an eye with myopia and positive diopter value (such as +3D) signifies an eye with hyperopia.

diplopia Condition in which a single object is perceived as two; also called double vision.

direct laryngoscopy An examination of the throat using a fiberoptic laryngoscope that is passed into the throat through the nose.

disease-modifying antirheumatic drug (DMARD) Any drug that actually reverses the disease process of an autoimmune disorder, as opposed to just treating symptoms.

disk Flexible pads of cartilage that separate the vertebrae from one another.

dislocation The displacement of a joint from its normal position.

diuresis Removal of fluid from the lungs.

diuretics Drugs that act on the kidneys to promote the excretion of excess water in the body.

diverticula (singular *diverticulum*) Small, balloon-like pockets that protrude through the muscular layer of the colon.

diverticular disease A disorder of the large intestine characterized by diverticula that protrude through the muscular layer of the colon.

diverticulitis An inflammation of diverticula in the colon.

diverticulosis The presence of diverticula in the colon.

Dix-Hallpike maneuver A test that determines whether vertigo is triggered by certain movements of the head.

dizziness Physical unsteadiness, imbalance, and lightheadedness associated with balance disorders.

dopamine An important chemical that helps transmit the nerve signals that cause the muscles to make smooth, controlled movements.

dorsal Relating to the back or posterior of a structure.

dorsiflexion Bending toward the dorsal aspect, as the wrist refers to lifting the wrist up.

double vision Another term for *diplopia*.

Dowager hump Another term for *kyphosis*.

dressing Materials that cover and protect a wound from the environment.

dressing changes The process of removing old bandages from a wound and replacing them with new, clean ones.

Dressler syndrome A delayed form of pericarditis that may occur weeks after a heart attack or heart surgery because of antibody formation.

drusen Yellow waste deposits that accumulate under the retina.

dry macular degeneration A form of macular degeneration in which the cells of the macula slowly begin to break down.

dual-chamber pacemaker A pacemaker consisting of two leads (one in the atrium and one in the ventricle) to allow pacing in both chambers of the heart to artificially restore the natural contraction sequence of the heart.

dual-energy x-ray absorptiometry (DEXA) The formal name for a *bone densitometry test*.

Duchenne muscular dystrophy (DMD) A common form of muscular dystrophy in children and the most rapidly progressive form of the disease.

duct A passage or tube with well-defined walls for the passage of air or liquids.

ductal carcinoma in situ (DCIS) A form of breast cancer in which cancer cells start in the milk passages (ducts) and have not penetrated the duct walls into the surrounding tissue.

ductus arteriosus A blood vessel that connects the aorta and pulmonary artery.

duodenal ulcer An ulcer that develops in the duodenum.

duodenum The first portion of the small intestine nearest the stomach.

dura mater The thick, outermost layer of the meninges.

DVT (deep vein thrombosis) Blood clotting in the veins of the inner thigh or leg.

dysarthria A group of speech disorders caused by disturbances in the strength or coordination of the muscles of the speech mechanism as a result of damage to the brain or nerves.

dysequilibrium Any disturbance of balance.

dysesthesia A condition in which a disagreeable sensation is produced by ordinary touch, temperature, or movement.

dysgeusia Distortion or absence of the sense of taste.

dysmenorrhea Difficult or painful menstruation.

dysmetria The inability to judge distance, power, and speed of a movement.

dysosmia Distortion or absence of the sense of smell.

dyspareunia Pain in the vagina or pelvis experienced during sexual intercourse.

dysphagia Difficult or painful swallowing.

dysphasia Difficulty in the use of language without mental impairment due to a brain lesion.

dysphonia Any impairment of the voice or difficulty speaking.

dysplasia Abnormal changes in cells, which sometimes indicate that cancer may develop.

dyspnea Difficulty breathing.

dyspraxia of speech Partial loss of the ability to consistently pronounce words in individuals with normal muscle tone and coordination of the speech muscles.

dystocia Difficult labor.

dystonia Abnormal muscle tone of one or more muscles.

dysuria Difficult or painful urination.

E

ear The organ responsible for hearing and balance.

ecchymoses (singular *ecchymosis*) Larger blotches of discoloration caused by bleeding from the blood vessels under the skin.

echocardiogram A test in which ultrasound is used to examine the heart anatomy.

eclampsia The final and most severe phase of preeclampsia if left untreated, leading to seizures or coma in the mother or even death of the mother and baby before, during, or after childbirth.

ectopic pregnancy A pregnancy that occurs when the egg implants itself outside the uterus.

ectopy, *syn.* **ectopic beat** A disturbance of the cardiac rhythm frequently related to the conduction system of the heart in which beats arise from fibers outside the region of the sinoatrial (SA) node normally responsible for impulse formation.

eczema A skin disorder that is characterized by itching, scaling, thickening of the skin, and is usually located on the face, elbows, knees, and arms.

edema, *syn.* **swelling** Abnormal accumulation of fluid in body tissues.

effacement Thinning of the cervix in preparation for delivery.

efferent nerves Nerve fibers that carry sensory information from the central nervous system to the peripheral nervous system.

effusion A collection of fluid inside a body cavity, such as around the lungs.

ejection fraction A measure of the output of the heart with each heartbeat.

electrical burns Burns due to contact with an electrical current.

electrocardiogram (EKG or ECG) A procedure used to measure and record the electrical activity of the heart.

electrocautery Removal of a lesion by burning with an electrical current.

electroencephalogram (EEG) A procedure that records the brain's continuous electrical activity by means of electrodes attached to the scalp.

electrolytes Minerals that regulate the body's balance of fluids.

electromyography (EMG) A method of evaluating the health of a muscle by measuring the electrical activity generated by muscles.

electrophysiology (EP) study A minimally invasive procedure using programmed stimulation protocols via catheters situated within the heart to investigate the cause, location of origin, and best treatment for various abnormal heart rhythms.

elevation An upward movement.

embryo The name given to a developing baby from the time of implantation in the uterus until about the eighth week of gestation.

embryo transfer The process of placing the fertilized eggs into a woman's uterus.

emesis Another word for *vomiting*.

emphysema A chronic lung disease in which there is permanent destruction of alveoli.

encephalocele The herniation of brain meninges through skull defect.

encopresis When a child who has been toilet trained soils their clothes, usually without knowing it.

endarterectomy The removal of fatty or cholesterol plaques and calcified deposits from the internal wall of an artery.

endocardium The thin, smooth membrane that lines the inside of the chambers of the heart and forms the surface of the valves.

endocervical curettage (ECC) The removal of tissue from the inside of the cervix using a curet.

endocrine gland A gland that releases its secretions directly into the bloodstream.

endometrial ablation A procedure in which the endometrial lining of the uterus is surgically removed.

endometrial biopsy A procedure in which a sample of tissue is obtained through a tube which is inserted into the uterus.

endometrial cancer A cancer that begins in the endometrium of the uterus.

endometrial hyperplasia An abnormal thickening of the endometrium caused by excessive cell growth.

endometrial resection A procedure to remove the lining of the uterus (endometrium).

endometriosis A disorder in which endometrial tissue grows elsewhere in the abdominal cavity.

endometritis Inflammation of the uterus.

endometrium The mucous membrane lining of the inner surface of the uterus that grows during each menstrual cycle and is shed in menstrual blood.

endoscope A flexible tube with a light and camera attached that is used to examine the interior surfaces of an organ.

endoscopic retrograde cholangiopancreatography (ERCP), *syn.* **cholangiography** A procedure in which the endoscope, along with x-ray imaging, is used to evaluate and treat problems in the bile ducts, gallbladder, and pancreas.

endoscopic ultrasound An endoscopy used in conjunction with ultrasound imaging.

endoscopy A procedure that uses a very flexible tube with a lens or camera and a light on the end, which is connected to a computer screen, allowing the physician to see inside the body.

endosteum The membrane that lines the marrow cavity of bone.

endothelium The smooth inner layer of a blood vessel that promotes the flow of blood through the vessel.

end-stage renal disease (ESRD) A name given to kidney failure that is so advanced that it cannot be reversed.

enterovirus A group of common viruses that is a common cause of viral meningitis.

enuresis The involuntary discharge of urine usually during sleep at night; bedwetting beyond the age when bladder control should have been established.

ependymoma A growth in the brain or spinal cord arising from the lining of the ventricles.

epicardium, *syn.* **visceral pericardium** The serous membrane that covers the outer surface of the myocardium and the inner part of the pericardium that folds back on itself to form the pericardial sac.

epidermal growth factor receptors (EGFRs) A protein in cells that initiates a signaling process that triggers abnormal cell growth.

epidermis The outermost, or superficial, layer of skin.

epididymis A coiled tube in each testis that stores sperm until ejaculation.

epididymitis An inflammation of the epididymis.

epidural, *syn.* **extradural** A term meaning immediately outside the dura mater.

epiglottis A flap of cartilage in the larynx that opens and closes in order to direct food and liquid into the esophagus and protect the airway during swallowing.

epilepsy The neurologic disorder characterized by recurrent seizures.

epiphysis The expanded end of a long bone.

epistaxis Profuse bleeding from the nose.

epithelial carcinoma A cancer which begins on the surface of the ovary.

epithelium A specialized type of tissue that normally lines the surfaces and cavities of the body.

Epstein-Barr virus (EBV) A type of virus that causes pneumonia.

erythema Another term for *redness*.

erythrocyte A red blood cell.

erythrocyte sedimentation rate (ESR), *syn.* **sed rate** A test that determines the rate of speed at which red blood cells settle in a glass tube containing a specimen of unclotted blood.

erythropoietin A hormone that aids in the formation of red blood cells.

esophageal sphincter A one-way valve located between the esophagus and stomach that regulates the entry of food into the stomach.

esophageal stricture Narrowing of the esophagus that makes swallowing solid foods difficult.

esophageal varices Abnormally enlarged veins in the lower part of the esophagus that develop when normal blood flow to the liver is blocked.

esophagitis Soreness and inflammation of the esophagus due to infection, toxicity from radiotherapy, chemotherapy, or physical injury.

esophagogastroduodenoscopy (EGD), *syn.* **upper endoscopy** A procedure in which the endoscope is used to evaluate the esophagus, stomach, and duodenum.

esophagoscopy A procedure in which an endoscope is used to evaluate the esophagus.

esophagram, *syn.* **esophagogram** The portion of an upper GI series that examines the esophagus.

esophagus A muscular channel that connects the throat with the stomach.

esophoria Position of the eyes in an over-converged position compensated by the external eye muscles so that the eyes do not appear turned inward.

esotropia Position of the eyes in an over-converged position so that non-fixating eye is turned inward. One eye looks straight; one looks inward.

essential hypertension High blood pressure that has no identifiable cause.

estrogen A group of hormones secreted by the ovaries which affect many aspects of the female body, including a woman's menstrual cycle and normal sexual and reproductive development.

ethmoid sinuses Approximately 6 to 12 sinuses on each side of the bridge of the nose.

eumelanin Brown-black melanins produced by melanocytes, which contribute to iris color.

eustachian tube A short, narrow passage that equalizes air pressure on both sides of the eardrum.

eversion Movement of the soles outward so they face away from each other and toes face inward.

Ewing sarcoma A malignant tumor occurring primarily in children and adolescents that tends to develop in the upper and lower legs, pelvis, upper arms, and ribs.

exanthem Another name for a rash.

excise To "cut out."

excision Surgical removal of a part of the body.

excisional biopsy The removal of an entire lesion for laboratory analysis.

excoriation An area of the skin covered by a crust, or scab, usually caused by scratching.

excretory system Another name for the *urinary system*.

exocrine gland A gland that drains its secretions through ducts, or tubes, to the surface of the body or other sites.

exocrine pancreas The area of the pancreas that produces digestive juices.

exocrine tumor A tumor arising in the area of the pancreas that produces digestive juices (exocrine pancreas).

exophoria A position of the eyes in an over-diverged position compensated by the external eye muscles so that the eyes do not appear turned outward.

exophthalmos A condition in which the eyes bulge in appearance as a result of water retention.

exotropia A position of the eyes in an over-diverged position so that non-fixating eye is turned outward.

expectant management, *syn.* **expectant therapy** Close monitoring of a disease by a physician instead of immediate treatment.

extension Straightening motion of a joint to increase the angle between two adjacent segments.

extensor muscle A muscle that contracts to extend or straighten a limb at the joint.

external auditory canal The tubular passage of the ear leading inward to the tympanic membrane (eardrum).

external beam radiation High-energy radiation that is delivered from outside the body and focused on the cancerous tumor.

external fixation A procedure that stabilizes and joins the ends of fractured (broken) bones by a splint or cast.

external genital organs Those genital structures found outside the body.

external respiration The exchange of gases that involves air from the external environment.

external rotation The movement of a joint around its long axis, away from the midline of the body.

external urethral sphincter A collective name for the muscles that expand and contract and work in conjunction with the internal urethral sphincter to control the flow of urine from the bladder.

extra-articular Outside the joints (in RA, affecting not only the joints but tissues, muscles, and organs outside of the joints).

extracorporeal shock wave lithotripsy (ESWL) A procedure that uses highly focused impulses projected from outside the body to pulverize kidney stones.

extraction A method of removing unwanted skin lesions such as milia or comedones on the face. A small lancet is used to puncture the lesion and then an instrument extracts the unwanted debris.

extraocular muscles Three pairs of muscles attached to the sclera that help move the eye in different directions.

extravasation The leaking of intravenous fluids or drugs into the surrounding tissue.

extubation The process of being removed from the ventilator.

eye chart Technically called a Snellen chart, a printed visual acuity chart consisting of Snellen optotypes, which are specifically formed letters of the alphabet arranged in rows of decreasing letter size.

eyelashes Hairs attached to the edge of the eyelids.

eyelid Either of two movable, protective, folds of flesh that cover and uncover the front of the eyeball.

F

facetectomy The surgical removal of one of the facets; excision of a facet joint.

facet joint Each of four joints formed above and below and on either side of a vertebra. The lower bony projection of one vertebra meets the upper projections of the vertebra below it, forming facet joints.

falciform ligament The fold of tissue dividing the right and left lobes of the liver.

fallopian tube, *syn.* **salpinx** One of a pair of tubular structures that extend from the upper edge of the uterus toward the ovaries.

false vocal folds, *syn.* **false vocal cords** A second set of folds above the true vocal folds that do not have a role in vocalization.

falx (cerebri) An extension of dura between the right and left hemispheres of the brain.

farsightedness Another term for *hyperopia*.

fecal fat test A measurement of the fat contained in a sample of stool.

fecal occult blood test A test that checks for hidden blood in the stool.

femur The long bone of the thigh.

fern test A test used to determine whether membranes have ruptured.

fertilization, *syn.* **conception** When sperm and egg form what will become a human individual.

fetal heart rate The normal heart rate for a full-term infant.

fetal scalp electrode (FSE) A device placed just under the skin of the baby's scalp that is used to monitor the baby's heartbeat while still in the uterus.

fetus The name given to a developing baby from the eighth week of gestation until delivery.

FEV1-FVC ratio A comparison of the FVC and FEV1, expressed as a percentage.

fiberoptic laryngoscope A long, thin fiberoptic telescope used to examine the throat.

fibrillation A rapid and unsynchronized quivering of the heart muscle during which no effective pumping action occurs.

fibrillin Along with collagen, a protein that gives skin elasticity, tone, and strength.

fibroblasts A common cell type found in connective tissue that is used in artificial skin grafts.

fibroid embolization A minimally invasive technique that involves identifying which arteries are supplying blood to the fibroids and then blocking off those arteries, resulting in a lack of blood supply to the fibroids, causing them to shrink.

fibroids Noncancerous growths in, on, or within the walls of the uterus.

fibromyalgia A syndrome characterized by chronic pain, stiffness, and tenderness of muscles, tendons, and joints without detectable inflammation.

fibrosis The formation of scar tissue.

fibrous joints Joints that do not move.

fibula The lateral and smaller of the two long bones in the lower leg between the knee and ankle.

filiform warts Narrow, small growths appearing on the eyelids, face, neck, or lips.

filtration A process whereby plasma and dissolved nutrients are forced out of the capillaries into tissue fluid.

fimbriae A number of finger-like extensions of the fallopian tube that drape over the ovary.

fine-needle aspiration (FNA) A type of biopsy in which a thin, hollow needle is used to withdraw fluid or tissue from the body for examination under a microscope.

fistula An abnormal opening or connection between any two parts of the body that are usually separate.

fixation The immobilization of the parts of a fractured bone.

flare An acute period of increased disease activity, such as in lupus.

flaring A widening of an area, such as the nostrils. In pulmonary medicine, often dictated as "nasal flaring."

flat bones Thin, plate-like bones with broad surfaces, such as those found in the skull and ribs.

flexible laryngoscopy A visual examination of the voice box while the patient is producing sound with the use of a flexible viewing tube passed through the patient's nose to the back of the throat.

flexion Bending motion of a joint to decrease the angle between two adjacent segments.

flexor muscle A muscle that contracts to bend a limb at the joint.

Fluid overload An unusual amount of water retained by the body.

fluorescein An orange-colored dye used in fluorescein angiography to help identify and photograph the retinal blood vessels.

fluorescein angiography, *syn.* **retinal photography** A diagnostic test by which the veins deep inside the eye are examined. Fluorescein dye is injected into a vein in the arm and circulated by the blood to the back of the eye, allowing for visual examination of the retinal vasculature of the eye.

fluoroscopy A continuous x-ray beam that is passed through a body part being examined then transmitted to a computer monitor so that the body part and its motion can be seen in detail.

focal segmental glomerulosclerosis A condition resulting in scar tissue that forms some segments of the glomeruli in the kidney.

focused ultrasound surgery (FUS) A procedure that uses high-frequency sound waves to destroy uterine fibroids.

follicle A pit in the skin containing the root of a shaft of hair.

follicles Fluid-filled sacs in the ovaries, each containing an immature ovum.

follicle stimulating hormone (FSH) A hormone secreted by the pituitary gland to stimulate the growth of eggs in the ovaries.

folliculitis An inflammation of the hair follicles due to an infection or irritation.

fontanels Spaces between the cranial bones that are filled with fibrous membranes.

foramen A hole or opening that acts as a passageway for nerves or blood vessels.

foramen magnum The large opening at the base of the skull where the spinal cord enters.

foraminotomy Surgical enlargement of the foramen/foramina.

forced expiratory flow (FEF) A measure of the average rate of flow during the middle half of forced vital capacity.

forced expiratory volume measured in one second (FEV1) The measurement taken when the patient takes the deepest breath possible and blows into the console's breathing tube, but only the first second of the forced exhalation is recorded.

forced vital capacity (FVC) The volume of air that can be expired forcibly and quickly after the patient has taken in the deepest breath possible.

forceps Metal surgical instruments resembling tongs with rounded edges that fit around the baby's head to assist with delivery.

fourth ventricle One of four ventricles located near the brainstem.

fovea centralis, *syn.* **fovea** The center of the macula the point of the sharpest and most acute visual acuity.

fraction of inspired oxygen (FiO2) The amount of oxygen in each inspiration.

fracture A break or crack in the bone.

fraternal twins Twins produced by the simultaneous fertilization of two separate egg cells.

free thyroxine (T4) A hormone produced by the thyroid gland that helps to regulate the body's metabolism.

frontal lobes The largest of the four lobes, located at the front of the brain.

frostbite Injury to the skin and underlying tissues when the body is exposed to very cold temperatures.

frozen embryo transfer The process of using cryopreserved embryos during the in vitro fertilization (IVF) transfer process.

fulguration Destroying tissue using an electric current.

full-thickness burn Another term for *third-degree burn*.

full-thickness skin graft A graft that includes both epidermal and complete dermal skin layers.

functional disorder An abnormality that is caused by an altered way in which the body works, rather than by a structural or biochemical problem.

functional MRI An MRI imaging study that obtains images of the brain while it is actually functioning or performing a task.

fundus The furthest point at the back of the eye, consisting of the retina, choroid membrane, sclera, optic disc, and blood vessels, as visualized through an ophthalmoscope.

fundus The enlarged portion of the stomach to the left and above the cardia.

fundus The dome-shaped top portion of the uterus that lies above the entrance of the fallopian tubes.

fusion inhibitors A class of drugs to treat HIV, which work by interfering with HIV's ability to enter the body's healthy immune system cells by blocking the merging of the virus with the cell membranes.

G

gallbladder A sac-shaped accessory organ attached to the lower surface of the liver that absorbs bile and releases it to the small intestine when food is present.

gallop A tripling or quadrupling of heart sounds that includes three or four sounds that resemble the cantering of a horse.

gallstones Lumps of rock-like material that forms inside the gallbladder.

gamma camera A special scanning camera used during a stress test that takes pictures as thallium mixes with the blood in the bloodstream and heart's arteries and enters heart muscle cells.

gangrene Tissue death due to obstruction, loss, or diminution of blood supply to the area.

gas exchange The process involving circulation of oxygen through the blood for use by the body, and the conversion of that oxygen to carbon dioxide for elimination by the body.

gastric emptying study (GES) A procedure to evaluate the rate at which food empties from the stomach and enters the small intestine.

gastric ulcer An ulcer that develops in the stomach.

gastric varices Abnormally dilated submucosal veins in the stomach that develop when normal blood flow to the liver is blocked.

gastritis A peptic disorder that involves inflammation of the lining of the stomach.

gastroduodenoscopy A procedure in which the endoscope is used to evaluate the stomach and duodenum.

gastroenterologist A medical specialist who cares for patients with diseases and disorders of the gastrointestinal system.

gastroenterology The study of the series of organs in the body responsible for digesting food and extracting nutrients necessary to sustain life.

gastroesophageal reflux disease (GERD) A condition whereby an excessive amount of stomach acids and enzymes flow backward from the stomach into the lower esophagus.

gastrointestinal (GI) system, *syn.* **alimentary canal** The system of organs in the body contained in a long coiled tube extending from the mouth to the anus that takes in food, digests it to extract energy and nutrients, and expels the remaining waste.

gastrointestinal reflux, *syn.* **heartburn** A painful burning feeling in your chest or throat that occurs when stomach acid backs up into the esophagus.

gastroparesis A medical condition consisting of a paresis (partial paralysis) of the stomach, resulting in food remaining in the stomach for a longer period of time than normal. Food then moves slowly or stops moving through the digestive tract.

gastroscopy A procedure in which the endoscope is used to evaluate the stomach.

gene Pieces of DNA which contain information for making specific proteins.

generalized seizures One of two main categories of seizures involving larger areas of the brain and often both hemispheres.

genital herpes A sexually transmitted disease caused by the herpes simplex virus.

genitals The external sex organs.

genital warts A sexually transmitted disease caused by the human papillomavirus (HPV).

genitourinary Referring to both the organs of male reproduction and urination.

genotype The genetic makeup of an organism or virus.

gestational diabetes A form of diabetes that develops during pregnancy.

giant cell arteritis (GCA), *syn.* **temporal arteritis** A form of vasculitis; an inflammation of the arteries that primarily supply the head.

girdles (shoulder and pelvic) The bones that support and attach the limbs to the axial skeleton.

glands A type of tissue that is made up of cells specialized for fluid secretions.

glans penis The external swelling at the tip of the penis.

Glasgow coma scale (GCS) A scoring system used to quantify a patient's level of consciousness following a brain injury.

glaucoma Painless disease of the eye characterized by increased pressure within the eye that can cause damage to the optic nerve.

glenoid fossa A shallow depression that forms the ball-and-socket joint of the shoulder with the humerus of the upper arm.

glia Non-neural (supporting) cells of the central and peripheral nervous system.

glioblastoma A rapidly growing tumor composed of primitive glial cells, mainly arising from astrocytes.

glioma A tumor that begins in the glial (supportive) tissue of the brain.

globus sensation The sensation of a lump in the throat.

glomerular capsule, *syn.* **Bowman capsule** A sac-like structure surrounding the glomerulus of each nephron of the kidneythat filters organic wastes, excess inorganic salts, and water from blood.

glomerular filtrate The filtered fluid from the glomeruli.

glomerular filtration rate (GFR) The rate at which wastes are filtered out of the blood per minute.

glomerulonephritis A type of glomerular kidney disease in which the kidneys' filters become inflamed and scarred, and slowly lose their ability to remove wastes and excess fluid from the blood to make urine.

glomerulosclerosis The term used to describe scarring that occurs within the kidneys in the small balls of tiny blood vessels called the glomeruli. The glomeruli assist the kidneys in filtering urine from the blood.

glomerulus (plural *glomeruli*) A ball-shaped cluster of tiny capillaries on a renal corpuscle, which is the area of blood filtering in the kidney.

goiter A mass on the neck that is actually an enlarged, inflamed thyroid gland.

gonio lens A special lens used in gonioscopic examination that indicates blockage or damage in the area where fluid drains from the eye.

gonioscopy A diagnostic procedure used to evaluate the angle between the cornea and the iris when testing for glaucoma.

gonorrhea A sexually transmitted bacterial infection caused by the organism *Neisseria gonorrhoeae*.

GPA system An abbreviated form of the terms gravida, para, and abortus used to indicate obstetric history.

grading The process of classifying cancer cells to provide information about probable growth rate of the tumor and its tendency to spread.

graft A section of vein, artery, skin or bone taken from one part of the body and transplanted to another part of the body.

granulocyte The most common type of white blood cell.

Graves disease An autoimmune thyroid disease caused by an overactivity of the thyroid gland.

gravida The total number of pregnancies a woman has experienced.

gray matter Another name for cerebral cortex because of its appearance.

greater saphenous vein A large subcutaneous vein located in the leg and thigh.

great longitudinal fissure The groove that separates the left and right hemispheres of the cerebrum.

great vessels A collective term to encompass the aorta, the superior and inferior vena cavae, and the pulmonary arteries and veins.

greenstick fracture A fracture in which one side of a bone is broken while the other is bent.

grunting A grunting noise heard during expiration during a lung examination.

gynecologist A physician who has specialized education and training in the health, disorders, and treatment of the female reproductive system.

gynecology The specialty of diseases of the female reproductive system.

gyri (singular *gyrus*) The name given to the folds of the cerebral cortex.

H

Haemophilus influenzae A microorganism responsible for pneumonia.

hard palate The anterior portion of the palate, or roof of the mouth, formed by bone.

Hashimoto thyroiditis, *syn.* **thyroiditis** An autoimmune condition that occurs when antibodies attack the thyroid gland directly, leading to insufficient production of thyroid hormone.

heart attack The death of heart muscle due to the loss of blood supply, caused by a complete blockage of a coronary artery.

heartbeat A single electrical pulsation from the heart muscle.

heart block A condition in which electrical impulses are not conducted in the normal fashion from the atria to the ventricles, leading to a slow heartbeat.

heart failure A condition in which the heart muscle does not pump the way it should. Right-side heart failure occurs if the heart can't pump enough blood to the lungs to pick up oxygen. Left-side heart failure occurs if the heart can't pump enough oxygen-rich blood to the rest of the body.

heart-lung machine A machine that provides circulation and oxygenates the blood while the heart is stopped during a coronary bypass procedure.

heart sounds The sounds associated with the heartbeat when listening to the heart through a stethoscope.

helper T cells T cells that communicate with other cells to organize and destroy foreign substances.

hemangioma A benign tumor of dilated blood vessels.

hematemesis Vomiting of blood.

hematochezia The passage of bloody stool.

hematocrit The percentage of red blood cells in the body. A low hematocrit is a sign of anemia.

hematologist A physician who specializes in disease of the blood and bone marrow.

hematoma A solid swelling of clotted blood within tissues.

hematopoiesis The process of formation and development of the blood cells.

hematuria The presence of red blood cells (RBCs) in the urine.

hemiplegia Paralysis of one side of the body.

hemodialysis A process of dialysis accomplished by the filtering of blood through a machine located outside the body.

hemoglobin A protein in red blood cells that transports oxygen and carbon dioxide and gives blood its red color.

hemolysis The alteration, dissolution, or destruction of red blood cells.

hemorrhage A leak of blood, or bleeding, from a vessel.

hemothorax A condition that results from blood accumulating in the pleural cavity.

hepatic ducts (right and left) The ducts that merge to form the common bile duct that carries bile from the liver into the duodenum.

hepatic flexure The name given to the turn of the colon next to the liver.

hepatic veins The veins connected to the liver.

hepatitis An inflammation of the cells of the liver.

hepatitis A virus, *syn.* **infectious hepatitis** The most common hepatitis virus, spread primarily by fecal-oral contamination or from eating contaminated food.

hepatitis B virus A form of hepatitis spread by blood and other body fluids.

hepatitis C virus A mild, slowly progressive form of the hepatitis virus that is spread by direct contact with infected blood or blood products, such as from blood transfusions (now rare), the sharing of IV drug needles or body piercing instruments, or even razors contaminated by microscopic amounts of blood.

hepatobiliary iminodiacetic acid (HIDA) scan, *syn.* **cholescintigraphy** An imaging test used to examine the function of the liver, gallbladder, and bile ducts.

hepatomegaly Enlarged liver.

herpes simplex A common viral infection of the skin or mucous membranes that causes blisters.

herpes zoster, *syn.* **shingles** A common viral infection of the nerves, characterized by a painful skin rash of small blisters anywhere on the body. It is a reactivation of chickenpox virus.

hertz (Hz) A measure of the tone of sound.

high-density lipoprotein (HDL) A type of cholesterol known as *good cholesterol.*

high-dose chemotherapy with stem cell rescue A procedure that involves harvesting of healthy stem cells, purifying and freezing them, and then infusing them back into the patient after high-dose chemotherapy has destroyed his/her immune system.

high-grade astrocytoma A glioma that occurs in the brainstem.

high-grade SIL Refers to a large number of precancerous cells on the surface of the cervix.

highly active antiretroviral therapy (HAART) The name given to multiple drugs used in combination to help suppress the HIV virus.

hilum Located above and behind the cardiac impression; a triangular depression. Part of an organ where structures such as blood vessels and nerves enter and leave the viscus. The area around the hilum is called "perihilar."

hippocampus The part of the limbic system involved in the formation and retrieval of memories and storage of dry facts.

hirsutism Excess growth of body and facial hair, including the chest, stomach, and back.

histamine A chemical that is released during an allergic reaction, causing symptoms in the eyes, nose, throat, lungs, skin, or gastrointestinal tract.

histamine-2 (H2) blockers A class of drugs that reduce the production of acid in the stomach.

hoarseness Abnormally rough or harsh tone to the voice.

Hodgkin lymphoma, Hodgkin disease A cancer that starts in the lymphatic tissue and is characterized microscopically by the presence of Reed-Sternberg cells.

Holmium laser A laser that operates in the infrared wavelength, producing a hot beam. It is used in surgical procedures involving the disintegration of stones and fibrous tissue.

Holter monitoring A procedure that allows for the continuous recording of electrocardiographic signals of the heart, usually over 24 hours, detecting and diagnosing changes in the heart's rate or rhythm.

homocysteine An amino acid used in cardiac risk factor testing.

horizontal gaze nystagmus An involuntary jerking or movement of the eyes that occurs as a person follows an object with the eyes to the side.

hormone A chemical substance released into the body by the endocrine glands to help the bod function optimally.

hormone therapy (HRT) The use of the female hormones estrogen and progestin (a synthetic form of progesterone) to replace those hormones the body no longer produces after menopause.

human chorionic gonadotropin (hCG) A protein produced in the placenta of pregnant women.

human immunodeficiency virus (HIV) The virus that causes AIDS by destroying the blood cells in the body that help the human immune system to function properly.

human leukocyte antigens (HLAs) Antigens tolerated by the body, corresponding to genes that govern immune responses.

human papillomavirus (HPV) A group of viruses that produce genital warts, transmitted through sexual contact, with some strains associated with increased instances of cervical and rectal cancer.

humerus The long bone in the arm that extends from the shoulder to the elbow.

hydrocephalus A condition, often congenital, marked by abnormal and excessive accumulation of cerebrospinal fluid in the cerebral ventricles. This dilates the ventricles and increases intracranial pressure.

hydronephrosis A condition that occurs as a result of urine accumulation in the upper urinary tract. This usually occurs from a blockage somewhere along the urinary tract.

hydrothorax The presence of water or fluid in the lung.

hyoid The single U-shaped bone that forms the larynx.

hyoid bone A horseshoe-shaped bone attached to muscles of the tongue and related structures, and to the larynx and related structures.

hyperacusis Heightened auditory acuity; the ear's hearing of abnormally loud sounds.

hypercalcemia An abnormally high level of calcium in blood.

hyperemesis gravidarum A complication of pregnancy characterized by severe and excessive nausea and vomiting.

hyperkalemia An excessive amount of potassium in the blood.

hyperlipidemia The general term used to describe elevated levels of cholesterol and other fatty substances in the blood.

hyperopia, *syn.* **farsightedness** An ocular condition in which light rays are improperly focused behind the retina resulting in blurred vision.

hyperplasia An abnormal increase in the number of cells in a tissue or an organ (i.e., cervix or the lining of the uterus).

hypertension, *syn.* **high blood pressure** A condition in which the pressure of the blood in the arteries is too high.

hyperthyroidism An overactivity of the thyroid gland, producing too much thyroid hormone.

hypertrophic cardiomyopathy Overgrowth of the heart muscle that can impair blow flood in and out of the heart.

hypertrophy A term meaning abnormal enlargement of a structure (such as the heart), which decreases blood flow.

hyperventilation A state in which there is an excessive amount of air entering the alveoli.

hyphema The presence of blood in the anterior chamber of the eye.

hypogeusia Diminished sensitivity to taste.

hypopharynx, *syn.* **laryngopharynx** The part of the pharynx lying below the aperture of the larynx and behind the larynx. It extends from the vestibule of the larynx to the esophagus at the level of the inferior border of the cricoid cartilage.

hypospadias A birth defect found in boys in which the opening to the urethra develops at a point under the penis instead of at the tip of the penis.

hypotension Blood pressure of less than 90/60 mmHg, usually because of loss of blood volume.

hypothalamus The part of the limbic system that regulates automatic functions such as appetite, thirst, and temperature.

hypothyroidism An underactivity of the thyroid gland, producing too little thyroid hormone.

hypoventilation A state in which there is a reduced amount of air entering the alveoli.

hypoxia Deficiency of oxygen supply to a tissue.

hysterectomy A surgery to remove the uterus and, sometimes, the cervix.

hysterosalpingogram (HSG) An x-ray study with contrast dye of the uterus and fallopian tubes.

hysteroscopy The visual examination of the interior of the uterus and fallopian tubes.

I

identical twins Twins conceived from one egg.

idiopathic cardiomyopathy A cardiomyopathy of unknown etiology.

ileal conduit A surgical connection in the abdomen that allows urine to bypass the bladder and exit into an external collecting pouch.

ileal pouch anal anastomosis (IPAA) A surgical procedure in which the colon and rectum are removed and an internal pouch is created from the end of the small intestine, which is then attached to the anus.

ileostomy A procedure that involves bringing the end of the small intestine out through a stoma in the abdomen.

ileum The end portion of the small intestine.

ileus An obstruction in the lower part of the small intestine.

ilium A major bony component of the pelvis.

imaging Tests or evaluation procedures that produce pictures of areas inside the body.

immune response The coordinated effort between the blood and lymphatic system to destroy invading microorganisms.

immune system A complex system of cells and proteins that works to protect the body from potentially harmful, infectious microorganisms, such as bacteria, viruses, and fungi.

immunocompromised An abnormal condition where one's ability to fight infection is decreased. This can be due to a disease process, certain medications, or a condition present at birth.

immunodeficiency A condition that is caused when the immune system fails to respond effectively to foreign substances that enter the body.

immunoelectrophoresis A test that identifies immunoglobins in a blood sample.

immunoglobulins A class of proteins produced and secreted by B cells in response to stimulation by antigens.

immunologist A clinician who specializes in the field of immunology.

immunology The study of the human immune system and the treatment of diseases involving that system.

immunosuppression When the body's immune system is weakened and is less able to fight infection and disease.

immunotherapy The artificial stimulation of the body's immune system to treat and fight disease.

immunotherapy agents Medications that work with the body's immune system to stop or slow the growth of cancer cells.

impetigo A bacterial skin infection characterized by microscopic pus filled blisters.

implantable cardioverter defibrillator (ICD), *syn.* **pacemaker** A small device implanted in the chest or abdomen that uses electrical shocks to help control life-threatening or irregular heartbeats.

implantable Collamer lens (ICL) procedure A surgical procedure whereby an ophthalmologist injects a specially formulated pliable lens into the eye that "unfolds" in the eye to correct nearsightedness.

impulse An electrical signal or action potential of a nerve fiber.

indirect laryngoscopy Also called a *mirror exam*, an examination of the throat using a mirror and light reflected down into the larynx.

infarction An area of tissue necrosis resulting from a sudden insufficiency of arterial or venous blood supply.

inferior vena cava The vein that carries blood from the body back to the heart.

infertility The inability of a female to become pregnant, regardless of the cause.

infiltration The leaking of fluid or medicine into tissues, which causes swelling.

inflammation Redness, swelling, heat, and pain in a tissue due to chemical or physical injury, infection, or allergic reaction.

inflammatory bowel disease (IBD) A group of disorders that cause the intestines to become chronically inflamed and swollen.

Infundibulum A stalk extending from the base of the brain to the pituitary gland.

infusion Delivering of fluids or medicines into the bloodstream over a period of time.

innate immune system The body's system of cells and mechanisms that provide an immediate defense against infection by other organisms.

inner ear The portion of the ear containing the organ of hearing and vestibular system for balance.

insemination The transfer of sperm to establish a pregnancy.

insertion The part of a muscle that attaches to a bone and moves when the muscle contracts.

instrumentation Metal supports sometimes used in orthopedic surgery. Common types of support include plates, rods or screws.

insufflation The process of instilling air or gas into a cavity (such as the abdomen).

integument The collective word for skin referred to by physicians.

integumentary system The skin, including its corresponding layers, derivatives, and all of its components.

intercostal muscles The muscles located between the ribs.

interferon A biological response modifier that stimulates the growth of certain disease fighting blood cells in the immune system.

interferon alpha A synthetically produced antiviral medication used to treat chronic hepatitis.

interleukin A biological response modifier that stimulates the growth of certain blood cells in the immune system that can fight cancer.

intermittent mandatory ventilation (IMV) A ventilator setting in which the ventilator delivers a set number of breaths each minute but allows the patient to breathe in between.

internal fixation A surgical procedure that stabilizes and joins the ends of fractured (broken) bones by mechanical devices such as metal plates, pins, rods wires or screws.

internal genital organs The structures involved in human reproduction.

internal respiration The exchange of gases between the blood in the capillaries and the cells of the body.

internal rotation Movement of a joint around its long axis, toward the midline of the body.

International Normalized Ratio (INR) A measurement of bilirubin and prothrombin time (PT) in the blood.

Interstitial cystitis A complex, chronic disorder characterized by an inflamed or irritated bladder wall.

interstitial nephritis An inflammation of the spaces between the renal tubules.

intertrigo A rash erupting in the folds of the skin.

interventricular foramen The opening through which the lateral ventricles of the brain communicate with the third ventricle.

intramuscular (IM) The injection of a drug into a muscle.

intraocular lens A permanent plastic lens that is implanted into the eye during cataract surgery.

intraocular lens implant (IOL) Permanent, artificial lens surgically inserted inside the eye to replace the crystalline lens following cataract surgery or clear lens extraction.

Intraocular pressure (IOP) Fluid pressure within the eye created by the continual production and drainage of aqueous fluid in the anterior chamber.

intrathecal Within a theca or the dura mater membrane that surrounds the spinal canal.

intrauterine pressure catheter (IUPC) A small catheter for measuring the strength and duration of uterine contractions, which is placed alongside the baby in the uterus.

intravenous (IV) The administration of drugs or fluids directly into the bloodstream.

intravenous immunoglobulin (IVIG) A pooled solution of antibodies compiled from the blood of many people, sterilized, and then administered to a patient with an autoimmune disorder.

intravenous pyelogram (IVP) A series of x-rays taken of the kidneys, ureters, and bladder to locate obstructions to the flow of urine using contrast dye.

introitus Another term for the opening of the vagina.

intubation The insertion of a tube into the patient's trachea to assist in the breathing process.

intussusception A type of intestinal obstruction that occurs when a portion of the intestine folds like a telescope, with one segment slipping inside another segment.

invasive cancer A cancer that spreads beyond its site of origin to involve other tissues and organs.

invasive (infiltrating) ductal carcinoma (IDC) Cancer that starts in a milk duct of the breast and goes on to invade the tissue of the breast.

invasive (infiltrating) lobular carcinoma (ILC) Cancer that starts in a lobule of the breast and goes on to invade the tissue of the breast.

inversion Movement of the soles inward so they face each other and toes face outward.

in vitro fertilization (IVF) A method of achieving pregnancy by artificial means.

involuntary muscle A muscle whose movement is controlled by the brain stem and spinal cord.

iridotomy Treatment for closed-angle glaucoma, usually done with a laser.

iris The colored part of the eye that controls the amount of light that enters the eye.

irregular bones Bones of varied shapes and sizes that are distributed throughout the skeleton.

irrigation-aspiration device A device used in cataract surgery that flushes lens debris with fluid and then uses suction to remove pieces of lens from the eye.

irritable bowel syndrome (IBS) A chronic disorder of motility of the digestive tract.

ischemia Insufficient blood flow to tissues due to blockage of the blood flow through the arteries.

ischium A major bony component of the pelvis.

J

jaundice The accumulation of bilirubin in the body resulting in a yellow color to the skin and whites of the eyes.

jejunum The middle portion of the small intestine.

joint, *syn.* **articulation** The point of connection between two or more bones, or between cartilage and bone.

J pouch An internal pouch created from the very end of the small intestine that is attached to the anus during an ileal pouch anal anastomosis (IPAA) procedure.

K

Kegel exercises A series of pelvic floor exercises that helps strengthen the muscles in and around the vagina.

keloid Firm, elevated scar tissue that extends beyond the normal scar tissue.

keratectomy Surgical removal of cornea l tissue.

keratin A tough, fibrous protein found in the epidermis, also found in the fingernails and hair.

keratinocyte The principal cell of the epidermis.

keratitis Inflammation of the cornea.

keratoconus A rare, degenerative corneal disease, in which the cornea thins and assumes the shape of a cone.

keratoplasty Surgical reshaping of the cornea.

keratotomy Surgical incision of the cornea.

kidney failure The loss of the kidneys' ability to adequately filter waste from the body adequately.

kidneys The paired organs of the genitourinary system responsible for the excretion of urine from the body.

kidney stone A hard, solid piece of material that forms in the kidney from crystals that separate from the urine and build up on the inner surface of the kidney.

kidney transplantation A surgical procedure in which a healthy kidney from a one person (the donor) is placed into the body of another person (the recipient).

kidney, ureter, and bladder x-ray (KUB) A supine x-ray of the kidney, ureters, and bladder.

killer T cells T cells that engulf and destroy all types of pathogens.

Klebsiella pneumoniae A microorganism responsible for pneumonia.

knee jerk The reflex tested by tapping the patellar tendon of the knee with a short, sharp blow to the tendon with a tendon hammer.

Koch (pouch) An internal pouch used to collect urine in a urostomy procedure.

KOH test A microscopic examination of the skin, hair, or nails for the presence of a fungus that infects these structures.

kyphosis A forward curvature of the thoracic spine caused by compression fractures.

L

labia Two sets of skin folds that serve to cover the female external genital organs and tissues.

labia majora A pair of prominent folds of skin from the mons pubis to the perineum that enclose and protect the other female external genital organs.

labia minora A pair of smaller folds of skin lying just inside the labia majora that surround the openings to the vagina and urethra.

labile Liable to change or easily altered; unpredictable.

labor The term given to the efforts of giving birth to a child at the conclusion of a pregnancy.

labyrinth The organ of balance located in the inner ear consisting of three semicircular canals and the vestibule.

lacrimal gland The gland that secretes tears.

lactation The production of milk in the breasts.

lamina The portion of bone that extends from the pedicle and curves around to complete the vertebral arch on the right and left sides.

laminectomy Removal of one or more entire lamina.

landmarks In otorhinolaryngology, particular patterns produced by the ossicles on the tympanic membrane similar to the position of a prominent or well-known object in a particular landscape.

laparoscope A specialized endoscope used to evaluate the interior of the abdomen, pelvic cavity, and other parts of the body.

laparoscopic cholecystectomy A minimally invasive procedure using the laparoscope and small incisions to remove the gallbladder.

laparoscopy Direct visualization of the abdominal cavity through a laparoscope, using a very small incision in the abdomen.

laparotomy Direct visualization of the abdominal cavity through a laparoscope, using a much larger incision in the abdomen.

large intestine, *syn.* **colon** A long, tube-like organ that moves waste material from the small intestine to be excreted by the body.

laryngeal paralysis The loss of function or feeling of one or both of the vocal folds.

laryngectomy Surgery to remove part or all of the larynx or voice box.

laryngitis Hoarse voice or the complete loss of the voice because of irritation to the vocal cords.

laryngopharyngeal reflux disease (LRD) A condition in which the flow of digestive acids from the stomach flow backward into the esophagus and into the tissues of the throat.

laryngospasm Closure of the vocal cords to prevent aspiration of acid into the trachea.

larynx, *syn.* **voice box** A tube-shaped structure situated at the top of the trachea, it is the organ of voice production and also serves a protective function for the airway.

laser in situ keratomileusis (LASIK) A procedure that involves correcting the shape of the cornea, and, hence, nearsightedness.

laser thermokeratoplasty (LTK) A procedure that treats hyperopia by shrinking the collagen in the cornea by means of a YAG laser.

lateral collateral ligament (LCL) The ligament that gives stability to the outer knee.

lateral meniscus The meniscus located on the outer side of the knee joint.

lateral ventricles A pair of ventricles in the brain where CSF is produced.

Lazarus sign A complex spontaneous movement by nerves in the spinal cord without conscious effort of the patient (such as after a patient is comatose or brain-dead).

lazy eye, *syn.* **amblyopia** An eye condition noted by reduced vision not correctable by glasses or contact lenses and is not due to any eye disease.

leads Electrodes on an EKG/ECG machine used to measure electrical impulses of the heart.

leaflets Flaps in the valves that regulate blood flow from the heart.

left anterior descending artery (LAD) A smaller artery that branches off the left main coronary artery.

left circumflex artery (LCA) A smaller artery that branches off the left main coronary artery.

left hemisphere One of two halves of the cerebrum that processes information.

left internal mammary artery (LIMA) A vessel located on the left side of the chest wall.

left main coronary The initial segment of the left coronary artery.

left ventricular dysfunction A heart condition in which the heart is unable to maintain normal cardiac output due to a deficiency in the left ventricle.

leiomyosarcoma A malignant cancer of smooth-muscle cells.

lens A clear, flexible structure located just behind the iris and pupil that allows for fine focusing of light as it passes through the eye.

lesion Any abnormal tissue found on or in an organism, usually damaged by disease or trauma.

leukemia Cancer of the blood.

leukocyte A type of white blood cell.

leukopenia Abnormally low levels of white blood cells in the blood.

leukotriene receptor antagonists A class of drugs that block leukotrienes, certain products of metabolism that cause narrowing and swelling of the airways in the lungs.

lichenification Skin that has thickened.

ligaments Bands of fibrous connective tissue that contain both elastic fibers and collagen.

limbic system A complex set of structures located in the cerebrum that are involved in emotions, moods, and some functions of memory.

limb salvage surgery A surgical procedure in which only the cancerous section of bone is removed but nearby muscles, tendons, and other structures remain intact.

lipase An enzyme produced by the pancreas that aids in digestion.

lipoma A benign fatty tumor usually composed of mature fat cells.

lipoprotein (a) A biochemical in the body measured in cardiac risk factor testing.

lithotripsy A method of breaking up urinary stones with a specialized tool and shock waves.

liver The largest organ in the body that plays a major role in the function of the body, including drug detoxification and the metabolism of sugars, fats, and proteins in the blood.

living-related transplant A transplantation procedure in which the donor is a living relative of the recipient.

lobar pneumonia An infection of the alveoli caused by fluid and pus filling an entire lobe of the lung.

lobectomy Removal of a lobe of the lung.

lobes Interconnected areas in the left and right hemispheres of the cerebrum that serve specific functions.

lobes of the liver The two sections (right and left) of the liver.

lobes of the lungs The four sections (right upper lobe, right lower lobe, left upper lobe, left lower lobe) of the lungs.

lobular carcinoma in situ (LCIS) Cancer that begins in the lobules of the breast but does not invade surrounding tissue.

lobules The glands in the breast that make breast milk.

localized A cancer that is still confined to the site of origin.

local transanal resection A noninvasive procedure whereby tumorous tissue is removed from the rectum.

long bones Bones that consist of a long shaft with two bulky ends or extremities.

loop electrosurgical excision procedure (LEEP) A procedure that uses a thin wire loop with an electric current running through it to remove cancerous tissue.

lordosis Curvature of the spine with the convexity forward.

low-density lipoprotein (LDL) A type of cholesterol known as *bad cholesterol.*

lower esophageal sphincter (LES) A valve-like structure that opens to let food into the stomach and then closes to keep the food and stomach acid from going back up.

lower gastrointestinal (GI) series, *syn.* **barium enema** An x-ray examination of the large intestine using contrast material.

lower respiratory tract The part of the respiratory system that includes the larynx, trachea, lungs, bronchial tubes, and alveoli.

low-grade SIL Refers to early precancerous changes in the cells of the lining of the cervix.

lub-dub The normal sound of a heartbeat.

lumbar Pertaining to the part of the back which extends from the lowest ribs down to the upper border of the pelvis.

lumbar diskography, *syn.* **diskogram** An enhanced x-ray of the intervertebral disks of the lower spine to determine if they are the source of a patient's back pain.

lumbar puncture (LP), *syn.* **spinal tap** A procedure used to evaluate the CSF from the space surrounding the spinal cord.

lumbar spine Lower spine, lower back; usually consists of 5 vertebrae.

lumpectomy A surgical procedure that involves removing only the tumor and some of the surrounding tissue of the breast.

lung cancer An uncontrolled proliferation of abnormal cells occurring in one or both lungs; also called *bronchogenic carcinoma.*

lungs Either of two respiratory organs in the chest that serves to remove carbon dioxide and provide oxygen to the blood.

lunula The white half-moon shaped part located at the nail base.

lupus anticoagulant (LA) An antiphospholipid antibody that causes damage to blood vessels and acts against proteins in the blood to promote clotting problems.

lupus flare A period of acute lupus disease activity.

luteinizing hormone (LH) A hormone secreted by the pituitary gland to stimulate the growth of eggs in the ovaries.

luteinizing hormone releasing hormone (LHRH) agonists A class of drugs that block the message from the pituitary gland for the testes to produce testosterone that enables a tumor to grow.

lymph A clear fluid containing immune cells that bathes tissues and organs throughout the body.

lymphadenectomy Surgical removal of lymph nodes.

lymphangioma A raised, yellow, tan, or red mark in the skin made up of enlarged lymphatic vessels.

lymphatic system The tissues and organs (including lymph nodes, spleen, thymus, and bone marrow) that produce and store lymphocytes (cells that fight infection) and the channels that carry the lymph fluid.

lymphedema Swelling caused by the obstruction of the lymphatic vessels.

lymph nodes Small, bean-shaped structures in the lymph vessels, which act as filters, collecting bacteria or cancer cells that may travel through the lymphatic system.

lymphocytes A type of white blood cell that helps the body fight infection.

lymphoid organs The name given to the organs of the immune system.

lymphoma A general term for a group of cancers that originate in the lymphocytes.

M

macrophage A type of specialized cell produced by the bone marrow, which quickly appears at the site of infection to ingest and destroy foreign particles.

macula The center area of the retina responsible for central vision, seeing color, and distinguishing fine detail.

macular degeneration A disease of the macula that results in the loss of central vision.

macular edema Collection of fluid in and under the macular portion of the retina.

macule The smaller version of a patch a flat discolored spot maculopapular A term that describes a lesion that contains both macules and papules.

magnetic resonance angiography (MRA) A test that uses a combination of a large magnet, radiofrequencies, and computer technology to obtain images of blood vessels in and around the neck and brain.

magnetic resonance cholangiopancreatography (MRCP) Similar to ERCP, except images are obtained using the MRI rather than x-ray.

magnetic resonance imaging (MRI) A diagnostic procedure that uses a combination of large magnets, radiofrequencies, and a computer to produce detailed images of organs and structures within the body.

malabsorption A condition in which the intestinal tract cannot digest fats as well as it should.

malignant Another term for *cancerous.*

malignant melanoma A rare, but sometimes deadly, skin cancer that begins as a mole that turns cancerous.

malignant tumor A cancerous growth with a tendency to invade and destroy nearby tissue and spread to other parts of the body.

malleus One of three ossicles of the middle ear, shaped like a hammer.

mammary glands Modified sweat glands located in the breasts that prepare for milk production during pregnancy.

mammogram An x-ray of the breasts.

mandible The lower jawbone.

marrow The spongy connective tissue within the cavities of the bones that produces many of the blood elements—red blood cells, white blood cells, and platelets—in the body.

mastectomy The surgical removal of all or part of the breast.

mastication The process of crushing and grinding of food by the teeth.

mastoid The back portion of the temporal bone behind the ear.

mastoid process The bone located behind the ear.

meatus The opening to the urethra.

mechanical ventilation The use of a machine to mechanically assist patients breathing when spontaneous breathing is absent or insufficient.

medial collateral ligament (MCL) The ligament that gives stability to the inner knee.

medial meniscus The meniscus located on the inner side of the knee joint.

median nerve The nerve formed from the brachial plexus that supplies muscles in the anterior forearm and thumb, as well as, sensation of the hand.

mediastinum The area of the body that contains the heart, the trachea, the esophagus, the thymus, and the lymph nodes.

medullary cavity, *syn.* **marrow cavity** The central area of the bone shaft of a long bone that contains bone marrow.

medulloblastoma, *syn.* **primitive neuroectodermal tumor (PNET)** A tumor that develops from the primitive (developing) nerve cells that normally do not remain in the body after birth.

meibomian glands Glands in the eyelids that secrete oils that lubricate the eyelids.

melanin The pigment responsible for absorbing ultraviolet light and giving skin its dark appearance.

melanocytes Pigment producing cells found in the basal layer of the skin.

melanoma A dangerous skin cancer that arises from the melanocytes in the epidermis.

melena Passage of black, tarry stools due to bleeding in the digestive system.

membrane A thin, flexible film of proteins and lipids that encloses the contents of a cell; it controls the substances that go into and come out of the cell. Also, a thin layer of tissue that covers the surface or lines the cavity of an organ.

memory T cells T cells that are created when they are exposed to a pathogen, remaining inactive until the same pathogen re-enters the body, at which time they remember the pathogen and reactivate to destroy it.

menarche The name given to a young woman's first menstrual period.

Ménière disease An inner ear disorder that can affect both hearing and balance.

meninges The three membranes covering the spinal cord and brain called the dura mater, arachnoid mater and pia mater.

meningioma A firm tumor arising from the meninges of the brain or spinal cord.

meningitis An inflammation or infection of the meninges.

meningocele A protrusion of the meninges of the spinal cord through a defect in the spinal column.

meniscectomy The surgical excision of meniscus, usually from a knee joint.

meniscus (plural *menisci*) One of two crescent-shaped disks of connective tissue between the bones of the knees that acts as shock absorber to cushion the lower part of the leg from the weight of the rest of the body.

menometrorrhagia Bleeding that occurs both during menses and at irregular intervals.

menopause The period preceding and following the last menstrual flow in a woman's life.

menorrhagia Heavy and prolonged uterine bleeding.

menses The menstrual flow.

menstrual cycle The series of changes a woman's body goes through to make eggs available for fertilization in preparation for possible pregnancy.

menstruation The periodic shedding of the uterine lining when no pregnancy occurs.

mesothelioma A rare form of cancer in which malignant cells develop in the mesothelium, the protective lining that covers most of the body's internal organs and commonly occurs in the pleura of the lungs.

mesothelium The protective lining that covers most of the body's internal organs.

metabolic acidosis A condition in which the blood is too acidic.

metabolic alkalosis Excessive blood alkalinity caused by an overabundance of bicarbonate in the blood or a loss of acid from the blood.

metabolic equivalents (METS) The measurement of aerobic exercise capacity.

metabolism The rate at which the body converts food into energy.

metacarpals The five bones of the hand.

metaphysis The area where the diaphysis meets the epiphysis in a long bone.

metaplasia A process that occurs when the normal adult cells in a tissue transform into a type of cell that is abnormal for that tissue.

metastasis The spread of cancer from one part of the body to another by way of the lymphatic system or blood stream.

metatarsals The five long bones of the foot.

metrorrhagia Any irregular, acyclical, nonmenstrual bleeding from the uterus, or bleeding between menstrual periods.

microkeratome A surgical instrument used to cut into the cornea and remove tissue.

microvascular clipping A procedure that involves cutting off the flow of blood supply to an aneurysm with the use of a spring-loaded clip.

microvascular decompression A microsurgical displacement of a blood vessel causing compression of the nerve root of the trigeminal nerve.

middle ear The part of the ear that includes the eardrum and three tiny bones of the middle ear, ending at the round window that leads to the inner ear.

millimeters of mercury (mmHg) A unit used to measure blood pressure.

miosis Pupillary constriction.

mitosis The basic process of cell division in which two identical cells are reproduced from a parent cell.

mitral valve The valve that links the left atrium and the left ventricle.

Model for End-Stage Liver Disease (MELD) A scoring system for allocating livers for transplantation in patients with liver disease.

modified radical mastectomy A surgical procedure that involves removing the entire breast as well as some of the surrounding tissues and structures.

Mohs micrographic surgery A technique of removing and examining a piece of tumor until the entire lesion is removed.

moles Small skin marks caused by pigment producing cells in the skin.

Mongolian spots Bluish black marks on the lower back and buttocks; affects mainly African American or Asian children.

monoclonal antibodies Laboratory produced substances that can locate and bind to cancer cells wherever they are in the body.

Monsel solution A substance commonly used in the dermatology office to coagulate blood after biopsies.

mons pubis A rounded mound of fatty tissue that covers the pubic bone.

morbidity Death as a result of disease.

motor nerves Nerves which carry commands from the brain and spinal cord to other parts of the body.

mucositis Inflammation of the mucous membranes.

mucous membrane The inner lining of the gastrointestinal tract, vagina, and nose.

multiple gated acquisition scan (MUGA) A test that uses technetium to evaluate the function of the heart's ventricles.

multiple myeloma A malignant tumor of the plasma cells of the bone marrow.

multiple sclerosis An inflammatory disease of the nervous system that disrupts communication between the brain and other parts of the body.

murmur An abnormal heart sound caused by turbulence as blood leaks past a defective heart valve.

muscle A type of body tissue responsible for the movement of the bones and joints.

muscular dystrophy (MD) A group of hereditary disorders characterized by progressive muscle wasting and weakness.

muscularis propria Another name for *detrusor muscle*.

musculoskeletal system The complex body system involving the body's muscles and skeleton, and including the joints, ligaments, tendons, and other connective tissue.

mutation Any change in DNA producing plasma cells.

mycologist A person who studies, identifies, and classifies fungi according to their microscopic appearance and in culture.

Mycoplasma pneumoniae The bacterial species that causes the disease entity known as mycoplasma pneumonia, also known as *walking pneumonia*.

mycosis A fungal infection of the skin.

mydriasis Dilation of the pupils.

myelin The material that envelopes neurons and helps neurons conduct electrical signals.

myelogram A specific x-ray study that uses an injection of a dye or contrast material into the spinal canal to allow careful evaluation of the spinal canal and nerve roots.

myelomeningocele A protrusion of the spinal cord and its coverings through a defect in the vertebral column.

myelopathy Any functional or pathologic disturbance in the spinal cord.

myelosuppression A drop in the blood counts caused by treatment, especially chemotherapy or radiotherapy.

myocardial band enzymes of creatine phosphokinase (CK-MB) A cardiac enzyme found in the cells of the heart.

myocardial infarction (MI), *syn.* **heart attack** Death of a portion of the heart muscle tissue due to a blockage or interruption in the supply of blood to the heart muscle.

myocardium The middle and thickest layer of the heart wall composed of cardiac muscle.

myoclonic seizures A type of generalized seizure characterized by repeated jerking contractions of one or more muscle groups.

myolysis A procedure in which an electric current is used to destroy the blood supply leading to a uterine fibroid.

myomectomy The surgical removal of a uterine fibroid.

myometrium The thick, muscular middle layer of the uterus.

myopathy Any disease of muscle.

myopia Also called nearsightedness or shortsightedness, the inability to see distant objects as clearly as near objects.

myotonic muscular dystrophy The most common adult form of muscular dystrophy, characterized by prolonged muscle spasms, cataracts, cardiac abnormalities, and hormonal disturbances.

myringotomy An opening made through the eardrum to allow fluid to drain from the middle ear and help equalize pressure in the ear.

N

nadir Commonly used in oncology, the term that is used when describing something at its lowest point, such as the lowest point to which white blood cell or platelet counts fall after chemotherapy.

nares (singular *naris*), *syn.* **nostrils** The two anterior openings located on either side of the nasal cavity.

nasal mucosa The mucous membrane that lines the nasal passages.

nasal polyps Fleshy outgrowths of the mucous membrane of the nose.

nasal septum A thin partition of cartilage and bone that separates the nostrils in the midline.

nasal sinus An air-filled, mucus-lined cavity within the cranial or facial bone.

nasogastric tube (NG tube) A feeding tube placed in the nose that runs to the stomach.

nasolacrimal ducts Two tiny canals at the end of each eyelid that drain tears into the nose.

nasopharynx The part of the pharynx that lies behind the nose and extends to the soft palate of the mouth.

nearsightedness Another term for *myopia*.

neck In aneurysms, the point where the aneurysm arises from the artery.

necrosis The death of most or all of the cells in an organ or tissue, or a part of an organ or tissue, due to disease, injury, or failure of blood to reach that area.

negative crossmatch A blood test result indicating that an organ transplantation should proceed.

neoplasm An abnormal growth that may be benign or malignant.

nephrectomy The surgical removal of the kidney.

nephritis A broad term for any inflammation of one or both kidneys.

nephrolithiasis The presence of stones in the kidneys.

nephrology The branch of medicine concerned with the study of the kidneys.

nephrons The microscopic filtering units of the kidney.

nephroscope An endoscopic instrument used to locate and remove kidney stones.

nephrotic syndrome A condition characterized by high levels of protein in the urine, low levels of protein in the blood, tissue swelling, and high cholesterol.

nephrotoxic Something that is toxic to the nervous system.

nerve conduction studies A test used in conjunction with EMG that measures the speed at which motor or sensory nerves conduct impulses.

nerve fiber A thread-like extension of a neuron that conducts electrical impulses.

nerve root The end of a spinal nerve nearest its attachment to the spinal cord.

nerves Structures of bundled neurons that conduct electrical impulses throughout the body.

nervous system The system of cells consisting of the brain, spinal cord, nerves, tissues, organs, and other structures that regulates the body's responses to internal and external stimuli.

neuralgia A paroxysmal pain extending along the course of one or more nerves.

neurectomy Excision of part of a nerve.

neuroblastoma A tumor of sympathetic nervous system origin, found mostly in infants and children.

neurofibroma A tumor of the peripheral nerves due to an abnormal collection of fibrous and insulating cells.

neurogenic bladder A disorder resulting from damage to nerves that govern the urinary tract.

neurologist A physician who specializes in the field of neurology.

neurology The medical specialty that deals with the diagnosis and treatment of diseases and disorders of the nervous system.

neuroma A tumor or new growth largely made up of nerve fibers and connective tissue.

neurons Nerve cells that carry messages to and from the central nervous system.

neuropathy Any functional or pathologic disturbance in the peripheral nervous system.

neurosonography An ultrasound examination of the brain and spinal column.

neurosurgery The discipline in medicine that focuses on the diagnosis and treatment of the nervous system.

neurotransmitters Nerve-signaling chemicals that send messages from one nerve cell to another.

neutropenia A condition of abnormally low levels of neutrophils in the blood.

neutrophil A type of specialized blood cell produced by the bone marrow that quickly appears at the site of infection to ingest and destroy foreign particles.

nevus, *syn.* **mole** A discoloration of the skin due to pigmentation that may be flat or raised.

Nissen fundoplication A surgical procedure in which the fundus of the stomach is wrapped around the lower part of the esophagus to prevent the backflow of acid into the esophagus.

nitrates A class of drugs that relieves chest pain by dilating blood vessels to increase blood flow to the myocardium.

nocturnal Pertaining to the hours of darkness or night.

nodule, *syn.* **papule** A small, elevated aggregation of cell on the skin.

nonalcoholic steatohepatitis (NASH) An inflammation of the liver caused by the presence of fat.

noncommunicating hydrocephalus A type of hydrocephalus that results from an obstruction within the ventricular system of the brain that prevents cerebral spina fluid from flowing normally within the brain.

non-Hodgkin lymphoma All lymphomas that originate in the lymphatic system that are *not* Hodgkin lymphoma.

non-small-cell lung cancer A disease in which malignant cancer cells form in the tissues of the lung.

nonunion A state of healing of the bone in which there is no healing.

normal spontaneous A vaginal birth without complications.

nulligravida Another term for *no pregnancies*.

nullipara Another term indicating *no deliveries of viable offspring*.

nystagmus An involuntary rhythmic shaking or movement of the eyes.

O

obstetrician A physician who is a specialist in the management of pregnancy and childbirth.

obstetrician/gynecologist (OB/GYN) A physician who provides medical and surgical care regarding women's gynecological health and also has particular expertise in reproductive issues.

obstetrics The branch of medicine that deals with the care of women during pregnancy, childbirth, and the recuperative period following delivery.

obstipation The inability for the colon to pass stool.

obtuse marginals (OM1, OM2) Lesser coronary vessels that branch off the left coronary artery in the heart.

occipital lobes Lobes located at the base of the brain that receive and process visual information and process events into visual memories.

occiput The back part of the head.

occlusion The state of closing or being closed, such as in vasculitis, a blood vessel that is closed off entirely, causing a blockage of blood flow altogether.

occult Another name for *hidden*.

olfactory Pertaining to the sense of smell.

oligodendroglioma A tumor that arises in the cells that produce myelin that covers and protects nerves.

oligomenorrhea Infrequent or light menstrual cycles.

oncogene A gene that normally directs cell growth, but when altered, can promote cancer.

oncogenesis The origin and development of cancer.

oncologist A physician who specializes in the treatment of cancer.

oncology The study and treatment of cancer.

onychomycosis A fungal infection in the nail.

oocyte An immature ovum contained in a follicle.

oophorectomy The surgical removal of one or both ovaries.

oophoritis Inflammation of the ovaries.

open cholecystectomy The traditional procedure of removing the gallbladder that involves a large surgical incision in the abdomen.

open fracture A fracture in which the bone is sticking through the skin. Also called a compound fracture.

open reduction Reduction by manipulation of bone, after incision in the skin and muscle over the site of the fracture.

open reduction and internal fixation (ORIF) The surgical repair of a fracture in which an incision is made to reduce the fracture, and instruments such as rods, screws, and plates, are used to stabilize the bone as it heals.

ophthalmologist A medical doctor (MD) or an osteopathic physician (DO) who is qualified and especially trained to diagnose and treat all eye and visual system problems, both medically and surgically.

ophthalmology The study of the eye.

ophthalmoscope A handheld illuminated instrument containing an angled mirror and various lenses to examine the internal structures of the eye.

ophthalmoscopy Examination of the internal structures of the eye using an illumination and magnification system.

opportunistic infections Life-threatening diseases that are caused by microbes such as viruses or bacteria that usually do not make healthy people sick.

opposition Movement of the hand where the thumb touches the fifth digit.

optic disc The region at the back of the eye where the optic nerve meets the retina, often called the "blind spot" of the eye.

optician An expert who designs, verifies, and dispenses lenses, frames, and other fabricated optical devices upon the prescription of an ophthalmologist or an optometrist.

optic nerve A bundle of nerve fibers that connect the retina with the brain responsible for transmitting nerve signals from the retina to the brain.

optometrist Eye care professional, graduate of optometry school, provides nonsurgical visual care. Specifically educated and trained to examine the eyes, and determine visual acuity as well as other vision problems and ocular abnormalities. An optometrist prescribes glasses and contact lenses to improve visual acuity.

orbit The boney socket containing the eyeball, fat, extraocular muscles, nerves, and blood vessels.

orchiectomy Surgical removal of the testicles.

orchitis An inflammation of the testis.

organ of Corti The actual hearing organ housed in the cochlea.

origin The part of a muscle that attaches to a bone and does not move when the muscle contracts.

oropharynx The part of the pharynx that lies at the back of the mouth.

orthopedics The science of diagnosis, treatment, rehabilitation, and prevention of diseases and abnormalities of the musculoskeletal system.

orthopedic surgeon (or orthopedist) The physician who diagnoses and treats injuries or diseases of the musculoskeletal system.

orthopedist A physician who manages the special problems associated with the musculoskeletal system.

orthopnea Breathing difficulty while lying down.

orthostatic hypotension The sudden temporary decrease in systolic blood pressure that occurs when a person changes position, resulting in a feeling of lightheadedness.

orthotics A support, brace, or splint used to support, align, prevent, or correct the function of movable parts of the body

oscilloscope A device that produces a visual trace of a voltage on a monitor during an EMG study.

ossicular chain The term that collectively describes the three movable bones of the middle ear.

osteoarthritis, *syn.* **degenerative joint disease (DJD)** A type of arthritis caused by inflammation, breakdown, and eventual loss of cartilage in the joints.

osteoblasts Bone cells (osteocytes) involved in the redepositing of new bone tissue in areas of old or damaged bone in the process of remodeling.

osteochondroma A benign tumor that contains both bone and cartilage, usually occurring near the end of a long bone, which takes the form of a cartilage-capped bony spur or outgrowth on the surface of the bone.

osteoclasts Bone cells (osteocytes) that break down old or damaged bone in the process of remodeling.

osteocytes A type of cell found in bone involved in the restructuring processes that regulate bone mass.

osteology The study of bones.

osteomyelitis Inflammation of bone due to infection, which may be localized or generalized.

osteonecrosis Death of bone tissue.

osteophytectomy Surgical removal of osteophytes (bony outgrowths) that may develop on the upper and/or lower edges of the vertebral bodies, often causing pressure on the spinal cord.

osteophytes A bony outgrowth or protuberance.

osteoporosis A condition that develops when bone is no longer replaced as quickly as it is removed, causing it to become weak and brittle.

osteosarcoma A fast-growing malignant tumor of the bone-forming cells.

osteotomy A process of cutting and reshaping a bone to reduce stress on an affected area in patients with avascular necrosis (AVN).

ostium The openings from each paranasal sinus to the nose.

ostomy bag A container attached to a stoma in the abdomen that collects the contents of the small intestine and unformed waste after an ileostomy procedure.

otitis externa The inflammation of the outer part of the ear extending to the auditory canal.

otitis media The inflammation of the middle ear caused by infection.

otolaryngologist, *syn.* **otorhinolaryngologist** A physician who specializes in diseases of the ears, nose, and throat.

otolaryngology, *syn.* **otorhinolaryngology** The study of the diseases and disorders of the ears, nose, and throat.

otosclerosis An abnormal growth of bone in the inner ear that prevents structures within the ear from working properly, resulting in a gradual loss of hearing.

outer ear The external portion of the ear, consisting of the pinna, or auricle, and the ear canal.

ova and parasites (O&P) A test that checks a stool sample for parasites or eggs (ova) associated with intestinal infections.

oval window The thin membrane that covers the opening to the inner ear.

ovarian cancer A cancer that forms in the cells of the ovary.

ovaries A pair of oval structures attached to the uterus, which produce hormones and release eggs (ova).

ovulation The process of discharging one ovum from an ovary.

ovulation induction The use of hormone therapy to stimulate the development of mature eggs.

ovum An egg cell in females that, if fertilized, can produce a human offspring.

oxygen saturation The amount of oxygen in the blood.

oxytocin A natural hormone produced by the pituitary gland that causes uterine contractions.

P

pacemaker, *syn.* **implantable cardioverter defibrillator (ICD)** A small device implanted in the chest or abdomen to help control abnormal heart rhythms.

palate The roof of the mouth.

palliate "To relieve, but not to cure," such as when chemotherapy is used to relieve the symptoms of cancer.

palliative treatment Treatment that relieves pain and other symptoms of disease but does not cure the disease.

pallor A paleness or decrease or absence of color in the skin.

palmar erythema A condition in which the palms of the hands may be reddish and blotchy.

pancolitis Ulcerative colitis that affects the entire colon.

pancreas A large gland that lies in front of the upper spine and behind the stomach, which allows digestive enzymes to flow into the duodenum.

pancreatic cancer A disease in which cancerous cells are found in the tissues of the pancreas.

pancreatic duct The duct that joins the pancreas to the small intestine.

pancreatitis Inflammation of the pancreas.

Pap smear A test that involves the microscopic examination of cells collected from the cervix to evaluate for abnormal cell changes.

papilla The tip of the renal pyramid.

papillary layer A thin layer of the dermis that connects to the epidermis.

papillary muscles Small muscles within the heart that anchor the heart valves.

papillary serous carcinoma A type of cancer that can originate in the uterus or the ovary.

papilledema Noninflammatory swelling/elevation of the optic nerve often due to increased intracranial pressure or space-occupying tumor.

papilloma A benign epithelial tumor, such as a genital wart.

Papillomavirus The virus that causes verrucae, or warts, in humans.

para The number of births of viable offspring.

paracentesis Removal of fluid from the abdomen by inserting a small needle through the skin.

paraplegia Paralysis of the lower part of the body including the legs.

parenchyma The essential or functional elements of an organ, as distinguished from its stroma or framework.

paresthesia Numbness, tingling, or a "pins and needles" feeling in the skin.

parietal layer Outer layer of the pleura.

parietal lobes The lobes located behind the frontal lobes, which interpret sensory information from the body associated with somatosensory functions, sense of direction, and problem-solving skills.

Parkinson disease A motor system disorder caused by deterioration of nerve cells in the brain that control body movement.

paronychia A bacterial infection caused by a tear in the skin at the side or base of a fingernail or toenail.

parotid (glands) A pair of salivary glands located at the side of the face and in front of and below the external ear.

paroxysmal Pertaining to the sudden onset of a symptom.

paroxysmal atrial tachycardia A rapid heart rate that starts and stops suddenly and unpredictably.

paroxysmal nocturnal dyspnea (PND) Difficulty breathing experienced when lying down, which is caused by lung congestion that results from partial heart failure and occurs suddenly at night.

partial hysterectomy The surgical removal of the uterus only.

partial nephrectomy Surgery to remove the kidney; only the part of the kidney that contains the tumor is removed.

partial pressure of carbon dioxide (PCO_2) The value of how well carbon dioxide is able to move out of the blood into the airspace of the lungs and out with exhaled air.

partial pressure of oxygen (PO_2) The overall content of oxygen in the blood and how well oxygen is able to move from the blood into the airspace of the lungs.

partial seizures One of two main categories of seizures that begin in a particular area of the brain.

partial-thickness burn Another term for *second-degree burn*.

passive immunity The immunity provided when a person is given antibodies to a disease rather than producing them through his or her own immune system.

passive motion Movement of a patient's joint by a person who is examining or treating the patient.

patella The kneecap.

patent Another word for *open*.

patent ductus arteriosus (PDA) A condition in which there is abnormal circulation of blood between the aorta and pulmonary artery.

pathogen Microorganisms that cause disease.

pathologic fracture A break in a bone that has been weakened by cancer or some disease condition.

pathologist A doctor who specializes in the diagnosis and classification of diseases by laboratory tests such as examination of tissue and cells under a microscope.

pathology The study of diseases by examination of body fluids and tissue.

pathways Routes taken by neurons to transport messages throughout the central nervous system.

peak expiratory flow (PEF) The rate of how fast air is expelled from the lungs.

peak flow monitoring A test that measures the rate of air flow, or how fast air is able to pass through the airways.

peau d'orange A symptom of cellulitis in which the skin resembles the tight peel of an orange.

pectoral girdles The bones that attach the arms to the axial skeleton.

pedunculated A term that describes something supported upon a stem or stalk.

pelvic examination An internal examination of the uterus, vagina, ovaries, fallopian tubes, bladder, and rectum.

pelvic girdle The bones that attach the lower limbs to the axial skeleton.

pelvic inflammatory disease (PID) A general term that refers to infection of the uterus, fallopian tubes, and ovaries.

pelvic lymph node dissection The removal of some or all lymph nodes from the pelvis.

penis The external male urinary and reproductive organ.

peptic disorders Gastrointestinal disorders that involve damage to the lining of the esophagus, stomach, or duodenum by stomach acids, enzymes, or infection with bacteria.

peptic ulcer A nonmalignant sore that develops in the lining of the stomach or duodenum.

peptic ulcer disease (PUD) A condition whereby a peptic ulcer develops in the stomach.

percutaneous nephrolithotomy (PCN) A procedure that uses a scope placed through an incision in the side of the abdomen to remove a kidney stone that is too big to pass.

percutaneous stereotactic rhizotomy A procedure in which the part of the trigeminal nerve in the face that causes pain is destroyed with a heating current.

percutaneous transluminal coronary angioplasty (PTCA) A procedure that opens narrowed arteries by using a catheter with a balloon on its tip.

pericardectomy The surgical removal of the portion of pericardium that has become rigid, compromising the function of the heart.

pericardial effusion A condition in which fluid accumulates in the pericardial sac.

pericardial sac, *syn.* **pericardium** A double-layered membrane that surrounds the heart like a sac.

pericardiocentesis, *syn.* **pericardial window** The drainage of excess fluid from the pericardial cavity with a catheter.

pericarditis An inflammation of the pericardium.

pericardium The membrane that surrounds the heart.

pericardium, *syn.* **pericardial sac** A double-layered membrane that surrounds the heart like a sac.

perimenopause The transition period of time before menopause, marked by a decreased production of estrogen and progesterone, irregular menstrual periods, and transitory psychological changes.

perimetrium The outer layer of the uterus that covers the body of the uterus and part of the cervix.

perineal Related to the perineum.

perineum The area between the anus and the sex organs.

periosteum Dense connective tissue that covers the outer surface of bone diaphyses.

peripheral blood stem cell transplant A method of collecting and freezing stem cells from the circulating blood-stream before chemotherapy, allowing the patient to receive higher-than-conventional doses of chemotherapy and/or radiation to destroy cancer cells. After completing high-dose chemotherapy or radiotherapy, the frozen stem cells are thawed and reintroduced to the patient via an intravenous infusion.

peripheral nervous system (PNS) The division of the nervous system outside of the brain and spinal cord, consisting of the cranial nerves, the spinal nerves, and the branches of those nerves.

peripheral neuropathy Damage to the peripheral nervous system (the nerves outside the spinal cord).

peripheral vision Ability to perceive the presence, motion, or color of objects outside the direct line of vision.

peristalsis Powerful wave-like movements of muscle that contract in syncopated pulses.

peritoneal dialysis A process of dialysis that involves using the peritoneum as a dialysis filter with which to filter the blood.

peritoneum The clear membrane that covers all the abdominal organs and the inside walls of the abdomen.

peritonitis A dangerous inflammation and infection of the lining of the abdominal wall.

pessary A plastic or rubber ring placed in the vagina to push the bladder back into place.

petechiae Tiny areas of bleeding under skin, usually due to a low platelet count.

Peyer patches A clump of lymphoid tissue located in the mucosa of the small intestine.

Peyronie disease A plaque, or hard lump, that forms on the erection tissue of the penis. The plaque often begins as an inflammation that may develop into a fibrous tissue.

Pfannenstiel incision A transverse incision made in the lower part of the abdomen during a cesarean section delivery.

pH A measure of the acidity or alkalinity of a solution.

phacoemulsification A process whereby the cloudy lens is removed from the eye during cataract surgery.

phalanges The bones of the fingers and toes.

pharynx, *syn.* **throat** A vertically elongated passageway that lies behind the mouth and nasal cavities just above the esophagus.

phonosurgery An operation that repositions or reshapes the vocal folds to improve vocal function.

phoropter A device that contains a range of corrective lenses for measurement of near-field and far-field visual acuity.

photocoagulation The focus of powerful light rays onto tiny spots on the back of the eye, producing heat, which seals retinal tears and cauterizes small blood vessels.

photodynamic therapy (PDT) A procedure that uses a photosensitizing agent, which is activated by exposure to light in order to destroy cancer cells.

photophobia Sensitivity to light.

photoreceptor layer The outermost layer of the retina where light is focused and converted into nerve impulses.

photoreceptors Microscopic light-sensitive cells that are located in the retina called *rods* and *cones*.

photorefractive keratectomy (PRK) A procedure to improve vision in which the surface of the cornea is reshaped using a laser device but without cutting into the cornea itself.

photoselective vaporization prostatectomy A procedure in which a high-power laser is used to vaporize prostatic adenomas.

photosensitivity Sensitivity to light.

phototherapy Exposure to ultraviolet light to decrease symptoms of some skin diseases.

physical therapy Exercises performed during the healing process and after the bone has healed, used to help restore normal muscle strength and joint motion and flexibility.

pia mater The thin, delicate membrane layer of the meninges that is closest to the surface of the brain and spinal cord.

PICC (peripherally inserted central catheter). An intravenous line inserted into the upper arm.

pinna, *syn.* **auricle** The external part of the ear.

pituitary An endocrine gland located in the limbic system, which produces hormones that control many functions of other endocrine glands in the body.

pityriasis A common skin condition characterized by scaly, pink, and inflamed skin.

placenta A temporary organ implanted in the uterus from which the fetus receives nutrients and oxygen from the mother's blood and passes waste.

placenta abruptio A complication of pregnancy in which the placenta breaks away, or abrupts, from the wall of the uterus too early, before the baby is born, causing premature birth or major blood loss in the mother.

placenta previa A complication of pregnancy in which the placenta is implanted in the lower part of the uterus instead of the upper part, causing it to partly or completely block the cervix.

plantar flexion Movement of the foot downward, away from the leg.

plantar warts Warts occurring on the soles of the feet.

plaques Fatty deposits that build up in the coronary arteries, causing the arteries to become narrow and to harden. In dermatology, they are raised patches of silvery scales commonly seen in psoriasis.

plasmapheresis A procedure of plasma exchange in patients with sudden, severe attacks of multiple sclerosis.

pleura A clear, shiny coating enveloping the lungs.

pleural cavity The body cavity that surrounds the lungs.

pleural effusion A collection of fluid or blood in the pleural space around the lung.

Pleur-Evac A water-seal suction device for pulmonary procedures.

pleurisy An inflammation of the pleura, the lining of the lungs and chest cavity.

Pneumocystis carinii The microorganism that causes interstitial plasma cell pneumonia in immunodeficient people.

Pneumocystis carinii **pneumonia (PCP),** now called *Pneumocystis jiroveci pneumonia* An infection of the lungs caused by the pathogen *Pneumocystis carinii (now renamed Pneumocystis jiroveci).*

pneumonectomy The surgical removal of a lung (usually to treat lung cancer).

pneumonia A serious lung disease in which inflammation, caused by bacteria and/or viruses, results in the accumulation of fluid and cellular debris in the air spaces of the lungs, preventing gas exchange.

pneumoperitoneum Air or gas in the abdominal cavity.

pneumothorax The accumulation of air or gas in the space between the lung and chest wall, resulting in partial or complete collapse of the lung.

polyarthritis Inflammation and soft tissue swelling of many joints at the same time.

polycystic kidney disease (PKD) A genetic disorder characterized by the growth of numerous fluid-filled cysts in the kidneys.

polyneuritis Inflammation of two or more nerves simultaneously.

polyp An overgrowth of tissue projecting into a body cavity.

polypectomy The removal of a polyp in the colon or rectum.

polysomnography, *syn.* **sleep study** A diagnostic test during which a number of physiologic variables are measured and recorded during a patient's sleep to help diagnose sleep disorders.

polyuria Excessive urination.

port wine stain A permanent flat, pink, red, or purple mark on the skin.

positive crossmatch A blood test result indicating that an organ transplantation should not proceed.

positive end-expiratory pressure (PEEP) A ventilator setting that maintains extra pressure at the end of expiration to help prevent the alveoli from collapsing.

positive pressure ventilation Provision of oxygen under pressure by a mechanical respirator.

positron emission tomography (PET) A nuclear diagnostic test that provides images of brain activity using radioactive isotopes injected into the bloodstream.

posterior capsule The thin membrane in the eye that holds the crystalline lens in place.

posterior chamber The larger, back section of the eye filled with fluid that nourishes the internal structures of the eye and helps maintain its shape and pressure.

posterior communicating artery (PComA) One of a pair of right-sided and left-sided arteries that connects the three cerebral arteries of the same side in the brain.

posterior cruciate ligament (PCL) The ligament, located in the center of the knee that controls backward movement of the tibia (shin bone).

posterior descending artery (PDA) The main branch off the right coronary artery.

posterior fontanel The area, sometimes called a *soft spot*, located towards the rear of the top of an infant's head between the growing skull bones.

posterior fossa A hollow depression in the back of the skull in which the cerebellum and several other structures are located.

posterior horn The back third of the meniscus in the knee.

postherpetic neuralgia (PNH) Chronic pain that lingers in the area of a shingles outbreak.

postmenopausal bleeding Any bleeding that occurs more than 6 months after the last normal menstrual period at menopause.

postmenopause The stage of menopause that begins when 12 full months have passed since the last menstrual period.

postnasal drip (PND) A condition in which mucus from the back of the nasopharynx drips down the back of the throat.

postvoid residual A urodynamic study that measures how well the bladder empties.

precancerous Abnormal changes in a cell that tends to become malignant.

preeclampsia, *syn.* **toxemia** A condition in pregnant women marked by high blood pressure and a high level of protein in the urine.

premature atrial contraction An extra heartbeat that originates from the atria before it should.

premature rupture of membranes (PROM) Refers to the sac of amniotic fluid rupturing before labor actually begins.

premature ventricular contraction (PVC) A contraction in the ventricle which occurs earlier than the next expected normal heartbeat.

presbycusis Loss of hearing that gradually occurs because of changes in the inner or middle ear in individuals as they grow older.

presbyopia The inability of the eyes to maintain a clear image as objects are moved closer, caused by reduced elasticity of the lens with increasing age.

presyncope A state consisting of lightheadedness, muscular weakness, and feeling faint but not actually fainting.

Prevnar A vaccine that protects against the seven most common strains of pneumococcal bacteria which cause invasive disease.

priapism Persistent erection of the penis because venous outflow is blocked.

primary brain tumor A tumor that originates in brain tissue.

primary hypertension A form of hypertension in which there is no identifiable cause.

primary site The place where cancer begins, usually named after the organ in which it starts. For example, cancer that starts in the breast is always breast cancer even if it spreads to other organs, such as bones or lungs.

primary tumor A tumor at the original site in which it first arose.

primigravida Another term for *first pregnancy*.

primitive Another word for *developing*.

proctitis A form of ulcerative colitis limited to the rectum.

proctocolectomy The surgical removal of the entire colon and rectum.

progesterone A female steroid hormone produced by the ovaries.

prognosis A statement about the likely outcome of a disease in a specific patient.

progression The spreading or growing of disease, with or without treatment.

progressive Increasing in severity.

progressive disease A disease that is increasing in scope or severity.

prolactin A lactation-stimulating hormone.

prolapse A structural abnormality in which the leaflets of the mitral valve do not close adequately.

pronation A turning of the forearm and hand so that the palm faxed downward.

prophylaxis Disease prevention measures.

proprioception A sense or a perception, usually at a subconscious level, of the movements and position of the body and especially its limbs, independent of vision but by input from sensory nerves.

prostate A gland in the male reproductive system just below the bladder that secretes prostate specific antigen (PSA), which helps form part of semen.

prostatectomy The surgical removal of part or all of the prostate gland.

prostate-specific antigen (PSA) An enzyme secreted by the prostate that helps form part of semen.

prostatitis An inflammation of the prostate gland.

prosthesis An artificial body part replacement.

protease inhibitors A group of drugs to treat HIV, which involves interrupting the ability of the virus to make copies of itself in later stages of infection.

proteinuria Excessive amounts of protein in the urine.

protocol The treatment plan which includes the drugs, dosages and dates for condition or disease.

proton pump inhibitors (PPIs) A class of drugs that reduce the production of acid in the stomach but that are more potent than H2 blockers and, thus, promote healing of ulcers in a shorter period of time.

protraction Moving a body part anteriorly.

pruritus Another term for *itching*.

pseudarthrosis Failure of fusion to achieve proper union of vertebrae.

psoralen A drug taken orally before exposure to ultraviolet light that lessens the effects of UV light on the skin.

psoriasis A chronic, recurring disease characterized by silvery scales called plaques on the skin.

pubic symphysis, *syn.* **pubic bone** One of three sections of the hipbone that form the front of the pelvis.

pulmonary artery The main blood vessel that takes blood from the heart to the lungs.

pulmonary circulation The part of vascular circulation that begins at the right ventricle of the heart.

pulmonary edema A buildup of fluid in the lungs.

pulmonary embolism (PE) A blockage of the pulmonary artery by foreign matter or by a blood clot.

pulmonary function tests (PFTs) A test with multiple values that measures the rate and volume of gas exchange in the respiratory system.

pulmonary hypertension Abnormally high blood pressure in the arteries of the lungs.

pulmonary perfusion Blood flow from the right side of the heart, through the pulmonary circulation, into the left side of the heart.

pulmonary stenosis A condition of obstructed outflow of blood from the right ventricle to the lungs.

pulmonary valve The outgoing valve of the right ventricle.

pulmonary veins The vessels responsible for carrying blood from the lungs to the heart.

pulse oximeter A small machine that displays the percentage of hemoglobin saturated with oxygen, anywhere from 0% to 100%.

pulse oximetry A noninvasive method of measuring oxygen saturation in the blood.

punch biopsy The removal of a sample of skin for laboratory analysis with a sharp, hollow instrument.

pupil The black opening or aperture in the iris where light enters the eye.

Purkinje fibers Specialized nerve fibers that help carry the electrical signals of cardiac conduction to the ventricles.

purpura Red or purple discolorations caused by bleeding from blood vessels under the skin.

PUVA therapy The combination of using psoralen and UV light as a treatment of certain skin diseases.

pyelonephritis An inflammation of the renal pelvis as a result of a bacterial or viral infection.

pyloric sphincter The circular layer of muscle around the pyloric opening that regulates the passage of food into the intestines.

pylorus The opening between the stomach and the small intestine.

pyuria The presence of pus in the urine.

Q

quadriplegia Paralysis of all four limbs.

R

radial keratotomy (RK) Outdated procedure once used to correct mild to moderate myopia, whereby making a series of spoke-like incisions around its periphery flattens the cornea.

radiation therapy (RT) The use of radiation to damage and kill cancer cells.

radical cystectomy A procedure in which the entire bladder is removed, along with part of the urethra and nearby organs and structures that may contain cancer cells.

radical retropubic (or suprapubic) prostatectomy A prostatectomy that is performed through an abdominal approach.

radiculitis Inflammation of the spinal nerve roots.

radionuclide scan An imaging scan in which a small amount of radioactive substance is injected into the vein. A machine measures levels of radioactivity in certain organs, thereby detecting any abnormal areas or tumors.

radius One of two forearm bones, located on the thumb side of the arm.

rales, *syn.* **crackles** Wet, crackling lung noises heard on inspiration, which indicate fluid in the air sacs of the lungs.

rash An inflammation in the skin affecting its appearance or texture.

Raynaud phenomenon A symptom of scleroderma in which blood vessels in the fingers become narrow, diminishing blood supply and causing fingers to become pale, waxy-white, or purple in cold temperatures.

receptors Nerve endings in the skin that sense pain, touch, temperature, and pressure.

rectum The lower end of the large intestine, leading to the anus.

recurrence The reappearance of a disease after previous treatment had caused the disease to disappear.

red marrow Bone marrow that actively produces blood cells.

reduction The realignment of bones back into their normal position.

Reed-Sternberg cells A kind of cell specific to Hodgkin lymphoma.

reflex A simple nerve circuit.

reflex sympathetic dystrophy A condition characterized by burning pain, abnormal sensitivity to sensory stimuli, poor circulation and changes in the skin, muscle, bone, and joints.

reflux nephropathy A condition in which the kidneys are damaged by backward flow of urine into the kidney.

refraction A process in which light is bent by the lens in order to produce a focused image on the retina. In optometry, an optical test which uses a device incorporating lenses of various strengths to measure near-field and far-field vision and to determine the corrective lens required for correction of such vision abnormalities as myopia or hyperopia.

refractive errors Disorders that cause improper focusing of the eye and subsequent blurring of vision.

regurgitation The leakage or backflow of blood into the atrium or the ventricle when the heart contracts.

rejection A reaction in which the immune system attacks foreign tissue, including transplanted organs.

relapsing-remitting multiple sclerosis A form of multiple sclerosis characterized by periods of flares of symptoms, followed by periods of remission.

remission Complete or partial disappearance of a disease; the period during which a disease is under control.

remodeling A continuous growth and replacement process of bone.

renal artery The artery that branches off from the abdominal aorta, which is the major source of blood to the kidneys.

renal calculus (plural *calculi*) A hard, solid piece of material that forms in the kidney from crystals that separate from the urine and build up on the inner surface of the kidney.

renal capsule The membrane that encapsulates each kidney.

renal columns The tissue of the renal cortex in between the renal pyramids.

renal corpuscle One of two major parts of a nephron of the kidney.

renal cortex The outermost area of the kidney.

renal failure Another name for *kidney failure*.

renal fascia A layer of connective tissue that attaches the kidney to the abdominal wall.

renal hilum The entrance on the medial border of the kidney through which blood vessels, nerves, and a ureter pass.

renal medulla The middle area of the kidney that contains the renal pyramids.

renal pelvis The large cavity formed by the expansion of the ureter within the kidney at the hilum that collects urine as it is produced.

renal pyramids Wedge-shaped masses of tissues in the renal medulla.

renal sinus The hollow cavity of the kidney.

renal tubule One of two major parts of a nephron of the kidney.

renal ultrasound A noninvasive test in which a transducer is passed over the kidney producing sound waves which bounce off of the kidney, transmitting a picture of the organ on a video screen.

renin An enzyme that initiates other enzymes that help raise blood pressure levels.

resection The surgical removal of tissue or part or all of an organ.

resectoscope A thin, lighted tube inserted through the penis into the urethra used to remove obstructing tissue and seal blood vessels in the prostate gland.

respiration The process of exchanging oxygen from the air for carbon dioxide from the body; includes the mechanical process of breathing, gas exchange, and oxygen and carbon dioxide transport to and from the cells.

respiratory acidosis A name given to a state in which there is a decreased amount of air entering the alveoli from hypoventilation.

respiratory alkalosis A name given to a state in which there is an increased amount of air entering the alveoli from hyperventilation.

respiratory failure Inability of the lungs to conduct gas exchange.

respiratory syncytial virus (RSV) A type of virus that causes pneumonia.

respiratory system A collective term for the organs and tissues involved in filtering incoming air, circulating oxygen to be used by the body through the blood, converting that oxygen to carbon dioxide, and eliminating carbon dioxide from the body.

restrictive cardiomyopathy A disorder in which the ventricles become stiff but not necessarily thickened, and do not fill with blood normally between heartbeats.

resuscitation, *syn.* **cardiopulmonary resuscitation (CPR)** An emergency procedure performed in an effort to manually preserve intact brain function until further measures are taken to restore spontaneous blood circulation and breathing in a person whose heart has stopped.

retina Layer of fine sensory tissue that lines the inside wall of the eye, composed of light sensitive cells known as rods and cones.

retinal detachment A condition wherein retina breaks away from the choroid membrane, causing it to lose nourishment and resulting in loss of vision unless successfully surgically repaired.

retraction Moving a body part posteriorly.

rheumatic fever An acute inflammatory disease involving the heart (as well as the skin, joints, and other tissues) caused by the body's immune reaction to a preceding streptococcal infection.

rheumatoid arthritis (RA) An inflammatory disease that involves the lining of the joint (synovium). The inflammation often affects the joints of the hands and the feet and tends to occur equally on both sides of the body.

rheumatoid factor (RF) An antibody found in the blood of most patients with rheumatoid arthritis.

Rh factor incompatibility A situation in pregnancy that occurs when the mother has Rh-negative blood and the Rh-positive blood, resulting in the mother's immune system producing antibodies to destroy the baby.

RhoGAM An injectable blood product used to protect an Rh-positive fetus from the antibodies produced by its Rh-negative mother.

rhonchi Abnormal dry, leathery sounds heard in the lungs, which indicate congestion and mucus in the bronchial tubes.

RICE treatment Acronym for rest, ice, compression, and elevation.

right coronary artery (RCA) A major coronary artery in the heart.

right hemisphere One of two halves of the cerebrum that processes information.

right internal mammary artery (RIMA) A vessel located on the right side of the chest wall.

right ventricular hypertrophy An abnormal enlargement of the right ventricle.

rigid laryngoscopy An examination of laryngeal structures with the use of a rigid tube that is passed through the patient's mouth.

ripening The term given to the softening of the cervix in preparation for delivery.

risk factor Anything that increases the chance of developing a disease, including a family history of cancer, use of tobacco products, certain foods or exposure to radiation- or cancer-causing agents.

rods One of the two types of light-sensitive cells, located primarily in the side areas of the retina that are responsible for visual sensitivity to movement, shapes, light and dark, and the ability to see in dim light.

Romberg test A type of test used to evaluate a patient's coordination and equilibrium.

rosacea A chronic inflammatory skin disease primarily affecting the face and around the eyes.

rub, *syn.* **pericardial friction rub** An abnormal heart sound that is caused by the friction between the beating heart and the pericardium.

rubor Another term for *rash.*

rubs Friction sounds in the lungs caused by inflammation of the pleura.

rupture of membranes The loss of fluid from the amniotic sac.

S

saccule One of three tiny organs of the vestibular system in the inner ear.

sacrum A curved triangular bone at the base of the spine, consisting of five vertebrae that have fused after puberty.

salivary glands Glands around the mouth and throat that secrete saliva into the oral cavity, where it is mixed with food during the process of chewing.

salpingectomy The surgical removal of one or both fallopian tubes.

salpingitis Inflammation of the fallopian tube.

salpingo-oophorectomy The surgical removal of a fallopian tube and ovary on either the left or the right side.

saphenous vein graft The harvested vein used in a coronary artery bypass graft (CABG) procedure.

sarcoma A cancer that starts in bone, muscle tissue, blood vessels, or fat tissues, and can develop anywhere in the body.

scalp The skin and membranous tissue covering the top of the head.

scapula, *syn.* **shoulder blade** A flat bone that anchors some of the muscles that move the upper arm.

schwannoma A tumor that begins in Schwann cells, which produce the myelin that protects the acoustic nerve.

sciatic nerve The largest nerve in the body. It extends from the sacral plexus, emerges from the pelvis and travels deep within the buttocks, then down the back of the thigh to the back of the knee, at which point it divides into the common peroneal and tibial nerves. The sciatic nerve supplies sensation to the back of the thigh, outer side of the leg, and essentially the whole foot.

SCL-70 A blood test that isolates the scleroderma antibody.

sclera The tough outer white layer that gives the eye its spherical shape.

sclerodactyly A symptom of scleroderma in which the skin becomes thickened and tight from loss of subcutaneous tissue.

scleroderma A chronic autoimmune disorder that affects the blood and connective tissue of the body, causing skin to harden and scar.

scoliosis An abnormal lateral curvature of the spinal column with rotation of the vertebrae within the curve.

scotoma An isolated area of varying size and shape, within the visual field, in which vision is absent or depressed; a *blind spot.*

screening Checking for disease when there are no symptoms.

scrotum A sac at the base of the penis that holds the testicles.

sebaceous cyst A blockage in a sebaceous gland causing a backup of fatty material.

sebaceous glands Glands that open into hair follicles and secrete sebum.

seborrheic dermatitis An inflammation of the sebum-rich areas of the skin of the scalp and face and occasionally the trunk of the body.

seborrheic keratosis A benign skin lesion occurring with the aging process. They appear on covered and uncovered areas of skin as raised rough spots. They may be light brown, brown or black. The color changes are harmless. These lesions do not need to be removed unless they itch, or become inflamed.

sebum An oily substance secreted by the sebaceous glands that softens and lubricates the skin.

secondary brain tumor A brain tumor caused by a cancer that originates in another part of the body.

secondary hypertension A form of hypertension in which another disease or medication is the cause.

secondary tumors Tumors that form as a result of cancer that has spread from other parts of the body.

secundigravida Another term for *second pregnancy*.

segmental cystectomy A procedure in which part of the bladder is removed.

seizure A sudden abnormal discharge of electrical activity in the brain.

selective estrogen receptor modulators (SERMs) A drug that acts like estrogen on some tissues without increasing the risk of hormone-related cancers.

self and non-self A concept that describes the ability of cells to recognize what belongs in the body and what does not.

semicircular canals One of three tiny organs of the vestibular system in the inner ear.

seminal vesicles Fluid-producing pouches that attach to the vas deferens near the base of the bladder, the fluid of which helps with sperm motility.

sensorineural hearing loss Hearing loss caused by an abnormality or defect in the auditory nerve or hair cells of the inner ear, preventing nerve impulses from being transmitted to the brain.

sensory nerves Spinal nerve roots that carry sensory information to the brain from other parts of the body.

sepsis Bacterial growth in the blood.

septoplasty A reconstructive procedure to correct a deviated septum.

Sessile A term that describes something with a broad base of attachment; not pedunculated.

severe combined immunodeficiency disease (SCID) A rare congenital disorder in infants resulting in a lack of all major immune defenses.

sexually transmitted A disease caused by a pathogen that is spread from person to person.

sexually transmitted disease (STD) A disease caused by a pathogen that is spread from person to person, primarily through sexual contact.

shave biopsy A technique using a small flexible blade to shave the surface of the lesion for analysis; typically used for superficial lesions of the skin.

sheath A thin covering that surrounds a tendon.

short bones Short, cube-shaped bones important for flexibility, such as those in fingers and toes.

shoulder girdle The bones that support and attach the arms to the axial skeleton.

shunt A silicone rubber tube used to divert CSF flow away from the brain to elsewhere in the body.

shunt revision A procedure that involves repairing or replacing a shunt.

sigmoid colon The bottom part of the colon after the descending colon and before the rectum.

sigmoidoscopy A shorter colonoscopic procedure used to investigate only the sigmoid colon.

simple mastectomy Excision of the breast including the nipple, areola, and some of the overlying skin.

simple partial seizures A type of partial seizure where there is no change in consciousness of the patient.

single photon emission computed tomography (SPECT) A nuclear diagnostic test that obtains images of blood flow to tissues.

singleton A term that refers to a pregnancy with only one baby.

sinoatrial (SA) node The "heart's natural pacemaker," a specialized cluster of cells located in the right atrium which initiates an electrical impulse that travels through the heart, causing it to beat.

sinuses The air-filled spaces inside the hollow bones of the skull.

sinus rhythm A normal cardiac rhythm.

Sjögren syndrome An autoimmune disorder in which the immune system attacks and destroys cells in the excretory glands, resulting in lack of saliva and tears.

skeletal muscle Muscle that is attached to the bones of the skeleton.

Skene glands A pair of glands located on each side of the lower end of the urethra.

skin The soft outer covering of the body and the site of the sense of touch.

skin biopsy The removal of a sample of skin for laboratory analysis.

skin graft A layer of skin taken from a healthy area on the body and transferred to an area with a skin defect or burned tissues.

skull The bony skeleton of the head.

SLAP Lesion Superior labral lesion in the shoulder.

SLE disease activity index (SLEDAI) A score derived from the level of activity of a lupus flare.

slit lamp An ophthalmic instrument producing a slender beam of light used to illuminate and examine the external and internal parts of the eye.

small bowel Another name for *small intestine*.

small-bowel resection A procedure in which a diseased portion of bowel is removed and the two healthy ends are joined back together.

small-cell lung cancer A type of lung cancer in which the cells appear small and round when viewed under the microscope and tend to spread quickly through the body via the blood.

small intestine A long tube that connects the stomach to the large intestine and is responsible for the actual digestion of food.

smear Any type of laboratory study in which material is thinly spread over the surface of a microscope slide for examination.

smooth muscle Muscle found in the digestive system, reproductive system, blood vessels, and some internal organs.

Snellen eye chart The most common chart used to test visual acuity with black letters of various sizes against a white background.

soft palate The posterior part of the palate, or roof of the mouth, formed by soft tissue.

Soft-tissue Generally, the ligaments, tendons, and muscles in the musculoskeletal system.

sonohysterogram (SHG) A visual study of the uterus and fallopian tubes using an ultrasound probe.

speculum An instrument with a curved blade used to spread apart the vaginal walls, allowing better visualization of the vagina and cervix.

spermatic cord The structure that carries sperm from the body.

sphygmomanometer An instrument that measures blood pressure.

spider angiomas Tiny clusters of red veins close to the surface of the skin.

spinal cord A long, tube-like column of nervous tissue that extends from the base of the skull to near the bottom of the spine, which carries both incoming and outgoing messages between the brain and the rest of the body.

spinal fusion An operative method of strengthening and limiting motion of the spinal column. Can be performed with a variety of metal instruments and bone grafts, or bone grafts alone.

spinous process A bony prominence projecting backward from a vertebra that can be felt under the skin on one's back.

spirogram A tracing that shows the values of expiratory volumes and flow rates.

spirometer A device that consists of a small plastic breathing tube hooked to a computerized console that records and prints the data it obtains.

spirometry A test that provides measurable feedback about the function of the lungs.

spleen The largest organ of the lymphatic system, which stores lymphocytes that assist the body in fighting infections.

splenic flexure The name given to the turn of the colon next to the spleen.

split-thickness skin graft A graft that includes the epidermal and part of the dermal skin layers.

spondylolisthesis Forward displacement or slippage (subluxation) of one vertebra over another.

spondylosis Degenerative bone changes in the spine usually most marked at the vertebral joints with bony spur formation.

spongy bone A lattice-like structure of bony tissue that makes up the inner portion of bone.

sprain An injury to a ligament resulting from a stretch or tear as a result of overuse or trauma.

spurs Bony outgrowths, or projections, from bones.

squamous cell carcinoma A cancer that begins in the squamous cells in the upper levels of the epidermis.

squamous intraepithelial lesion (SIL) A general term used to describe abnormal cells in the lining of the cervix.

squamous skin cells Flattened cells that make the skin waterproof and provide the main barrier to skin infection.

staging An organized process of determining how far a cancer has spread.

stapes One of three ossicles of the middle ear, shaped like a stirrup.

Staphylococcus aureus A microorganism responsible for pneumonia.

station The position of the baby's presenting part relative to the mother's ischial spine.

status epilepticus A prolonged seizure or series of seizures that last for more than 30 minutes, during which time the patient is unconscious.

steatorrhea A condition in which the feces contain excessive fat, causing them to float and be very foul smelling.

stem cells Immature cells that grow into different types of cells.

stenosis A constriction or narrowing of a duct or passage; a stricture.

stent A mesh-like metal tube placed in an artery to keep it open.

stereotactic radiosurgery A procedure that involves delivering a single highly concentrated dose of ionizing radiation to a target at the trigeminal nerve root.

sternum, *syn.* **breast bone** A flat, dagger-shaped bone located in the middle part of the anterior wall of the thorax that, along with the ribs, forms the rib cage.

steroids Drugs used to relieve swelling and inflammation.

stoma An artificially created opening.

stomach A muscular, sac-like organ that receives food from the esophagus during digestion.

stool Firm solid waste material excreted from the body.

stool culture A test that checks for the presence of abnormal bacteria in the digestive tract.

strabismus A condition that occurs when the muscles of the eye do not aligned properly and binocular vision is not present.

strain An injury to a tendon or muscle resulting from overuse or trauma.

stratum corneum, *syn.* **horny layer** The uppermost epidural layer.

stratum germinativum, *syn.* **basal layer** The bottom sublayer of the epidermis.

stratum granulosum A grainy layer of skin above the spiny layer.

stratum lucidum A thick, clear layer of skin that is particularly thick in the hands and soles of the feet.

stratum spinosum A spiny layer of skin above the basal layer *Streptococcus pneumoniae*. The most common bacteria that cause bacterial pneumonia.

stress fractures A fracture caused by repetitive stress, as may occur in sports, strenuous exercise, or heavy physical labor.

stress incontinence The most common type of incontinence that involves the leakage of urine during exercise, coughing, sneezing, laughing, lifting heavy objects, or other body movements that put pressure on the bladder.

striae, *syn.* **stripe or streak** A term describing the appearance of muscle fibers.

striated muscles Muscles composed of fibers that have horizontal stripes when viewed under a microscope.

stricture A narrowing of part of the intestine.

stricturoplasty A procedure used to widen narrowed areas of the intestines due to scarring.

stridor A whistling sound heard on inspiration that indicates obstruction of the trachea or larynx.

stroke An impeded blood supply in the brain, resulting in damage and death of large areas of the brain.

struvite A chemical compound that can form crystals in the kidney and bladder.

subacute A condition whose frequency lies between acute and chronic.

subarachnoid Located under the arachnoid membrane and above the pia mater.

subarachnoid hemorrhage A leak of blood into the space between the brain and the skull.

subarachnoid space The space through which cerebrospinal fluid (CSF) circulates in the spine.

subcutaneous A word meaning "beneath the skin."

subcutaneous layer The fat layer below the dermis.

subcuticular Underneath the dermis.

subdural space The space between the dura mater and the arachnoid membrane of the meninges.

sublingual (glands) A pair of salivary glands located under the tongue.

subluxation An incomplete or partial dislocation that separates a joint's movable surfaces.

submandibular (glands) A pair of salivary glands located beneath the lower jaw (mandible).

subpial resection A series of surgical cuts to help isolate the area of the brain that is causing seizures.

sudden cardiac arrest A medical emergency resulting from the cessation or inadequate contraction of the left ventricle of the heart that immediately causes body-wide circulatory failure.

sulci (singular *sulcus*) The name given to the grooves between the folds of the cerebral cortex.

superficial burn Another term for *first-degree burn*.

superior vena cava The major vein that carries blood from the upper body to the right atrium.

supination A turning of the forearm and hand so that the palm faces upward. The opposite of pronation.

supraventricular tachycardia (SVT) A tachycardia originating from above the ventricles.

surfactant Fluid secreted by the cells of the alveoli that reduces the surface tension of pulmonary fluids; it contributes to the elastic properties of pulmonary tissue.

sutures Immovable interlocking joints that join the skull bones together.

sweat glands Glands that produce sweat.

syncope Fainting, loss of consciousness, or dizziness which may be due to a transient disturbance of cardiac rhythm (arrhythmia) or other causes.

synovectomy The removal of inflamed synovial tissue from the joints.

synovial fluid A lubricating fluid that helps the joints more easily move.

synovial joints Joints that can move in many directions.

synovium A fibrous envelope that produces a fluid to help to reduce friction and wear in a joint.

systemic circulation The part of vascular circulation that begins at the left ventricle.

systemic lupus erythematosus (SLE), syn. **lupus** A multisystem autoimmune disease characterized by achy joints; inflammation of the fibrous tissue surrounding the heart; unexplained rashes on the face, neck, or scalp; and other disorders.

systemic scleroderma A more widespread form of scleroderma, initially affecting the skin and then gradually involving the esophagus, lungs, intestines, or other organs, causing them to function abnormally.

systole The part of the cardiac cycle in which the heart muscle contracts, forcing the blood from the ventricles into the main blood vessels.

systolic pressure The top number in a blood pressure reading that represents the maximum pressure in the arteries as the heart contracts.

T

tachycardia, *syn.* **tachyarrhythmia** Rapid beating of either or both chambers of the heart, usually defined as a resting heart rate over 100 beats per minute.

Takayasu arteritis A form of vasculitis that affects the aorta and its branches.

talus The bone of the foot that articulates with the tibia and fibula to form the ankle joint.

tamoxifen An anticancer drug used in hormone therapy to block the effects of estrogen.

tarsals The bones that comprise the seven bones in the ankle.

tarsus Connective tissue making up the eyelids.

T cells A type of lymphocyte that matures in the thymus, which detects invading bacteria or viruses and stimulates B cells to produce antibodies against them.

technetium A radioactive isotope injected into the body that is used to reveal abnormalities in the heart wall.

technetium 99 A radioactive contrast used in bone scans.

temporal lobectomy The removal of a portion of the temporal lobe that causes seizures.

temporal lobes Lobes located on the side of the brain that process memory, language, and music.

tendon The tissue by which a muscle attaches to bone.

tendonitis Inflammation of a tendon.

tension A name given to the balance of pressure in the eye.

testes (singular *testis*) Another name for *testicles*.

testicles The organs that produce sperm and testosterone.

testicular torsion A twisting of the testicles around the spermatic cord, resulting in decreased blood flow to the testes.

testis One of the pair of male gonads that produce semen; suspended in the scrotum by the spermatic cords.

tetralogy of Fallot A condition that causes insufficient oxygen levels in the blood.

thalamus The part of the limbic system that relays information that comes through the cerebral cortex.

thallium Radioactive material that is injected into a vein to show damaged areas of heart muscle.

third ventricle One of four ventricles located in the median cavity of the brain.

thoracic A term relating to the vertebrae of the chest.

thoracic cage The bones of the chest.

thorax The chest cavity.

three-pillow orthopnea A description of the patient's sleep habits in which the patient requires three pillows to breathe comfortably while sleeping.

thrombocytopenia Abnormally low levels of platelets in the blood.

thrombolytics A class of drugs that dissolve a clot that blocks blood flow through an artery.

thrombophlebitis Inflammation of veins with blood clots inside the veins.

thrombus A blood clot that forms in a vessel and impedes blood flow.

thymus A gland that produces mature T cells, found in the thorax under the breastbone.

thyroglobulin A protein produced by normal thyroid tissue.

thyroid A butterfly-shaped gland located in the neck, just below the larynx.

thyroid-stimulating hormone (TSH) A hormone produced by the pituitary gland that enables the thyroid gland to produce thyroid hormone.

thyroplasty A surgical technique to improve voice by altering the cartilages of the larynx.

thyroxine (T4) A hormone produced by the thyroid gland which helps to regulate the body's metabolism.

tibia One of the two lower leg bones.

tidal volume Indicates the amount of air inhaled or exhaled during normal breathing.

tinea, *syn.* **ringworm** A fungal infection of the skin resulting in a characteristic red, ring-shaped rash as it grows.

tinea barbae A fungal infection involving the beard area on the face.

tinea capitis A fungal infection involving the scalp or neck.

tinea corporis A fungal infection involving the hairless parts of the body.

tinea cruris, *syn.* **jock itch** A fungal infection involving the groin.

tinea pedis, *syn.* **athlete' foot** A fungal infection involving the feet.

tinnitus The sensation of a ringing, roaring, or buzzing sound in the ears or head, often associated with various forms of hearing impairment.

tissue A group or layer of cells that together perform specific functions.

tissue typing A test used to determine the genetic match between the donor of a transplanted organ and its recipient.

titer The concentration or strength of a substance in a particular solution.

tocodynamometer An instrument used to measure the force of uterine contractions.

tonic-clonic seizure, *syn.* **grand mal seizure** A type of generalized seizure characterized by a stiffening of the body and jerking body movements and sometimes loss of consciousness.

tonometer (Tono-Pen) A device used to calculate the pressure in the eye from the change in the light reflected off the corneas.

tonometry A procedure to test for glaucoma that measures the degree of intraocular pressure.

topical immunomodulators (TIMS) A class of drugs that inhibit inflammatory skin reactions when treating for symptoms of some skin diseases.

torticollis The spasmodic contraction of neck muscles drawing the head to one side with the chin pointing to the other side.

total abdominal hysterectomy The surgical removal of the uterus and cervix by means of access from the abdomen.

total hip arthroplasty (THA) A procedure in which a diseased joint in the hip is replaced with long-lasting artificial components.

total hip replacement A surgical procedure in which the diseased ball and socket of the hip joint are completely removed and replaced with artificial materials.

total hysterectomy The surgical removal of the uterus, including the cervix; the fallopian tubes and the ovaries remain.

total joint replacement, *syn.* **arthroplasty** A surgical repair or replacement of a diseased joint.

total knee arthroplasty (TKA) A procedure in which a diseased joint in the knee is replaced with long-lasting artificial components.

total knee replacement A surgical procedure in which damaged parts of the knee joint are replaced with artificial parts.

total lung capacity (TLC) The total volume of the lungs when maximally inflated.

TPAL system A system used to describe the obstetric history of a patient.

trabeculae Thin bony plates that make up part of spongy bone.

trabeculectomy A procedure to treat glaucoma where an opening is surgically created in the wall of the eye so that aqueous humor can drain.

trabeculoplasty A procedure to treat glaucoma where the laser is focused into the eye in such a way as to let aqueous fluid leave the eye more efficiently.

trachea A tube-like portion of the respiratory tract that connects the larynx with the bronchi.

tracheostomy A temporary opening created in the trachea, allowing air to bypass an obstruction.

traction A process of aligning bone with the use a gentle, steady, pulling action.

transcutaneous electrical nerve stimulation (TENS) A method of providing pain relief using electrical signals which are sent to the nerve endings.

transfer catheter A catheter with a syringe that is used to transfer fertilized eggs into the woman's uterus.

transitional cell carcinoma A cancer that originates in the transitional cells of the bladder.

transjugular intrahepatic portosystemic shunt (TIPS) A procedure used to treat bleeding from the esophagus or stomach and ascites in the abdomen caused by portal hypertension by inserting a stent to connect the portal veins to adjacent blood vessels that have lower pressure.

transposition of the great vessels A condition in which the location of the aorta and pulmonary artery is switched.

transrectal ultrasound An ultrasound procedure used to examine the prostate.

transsphenoidal Refers to a path going through the sphenoid bone located under the eyes and over the nose that a surgeon uses to gain access to the pituitary gland.

transsphenoidal approach An operative method of reaching the pituitary gland or skull base traversing the nose and sinuses.

transurethral hyperthermia A procedure that uses heat, usually provided by microwaves, to shrink the prostate.

transurethral laser incision of the prostate (TULIP) The use of laser through the urethra that melts the tissue.

transurethral resection of bladder (tumor) (TURB) A surgical procedure in which a tumor is removed from the bladder through the urethra.

transurethral resection of the prostate (TURP) A surgical procedure to remove tissue from the prostate using a lighted resectoscope inserted through the urethra.

transverse colon The top portion of the colon extending from the hepatic flexure to the splenic flexure.

transverse fracture A fracture in which the break is across the bone, at a right angle to the long axis of the bone.

transverse process The wing of bone on either side of each vertebral arch where the pedicle meets the lamina.

tricuspid valve The valve that links the right atrium and the right ventricle and prevents the backflow from the ventricle to the atrium.

trigeminal nerve The fifth cranial nerve and the largest. It is mainly sensory except for a small motor branch that supplies the muscles for chewing. The branches of the trigeminal nerve provide sensation to the eye and forehead, mid face, and upper and lower jaw.

trigeminal neuralgia, *syn.* **tic douloureux** A disorder of the trigeminal nerve causing sudden attacks of pain on one side of the face.

trigeminy A repeating pattern of two normal contractions of the heart followed by one premature contraction.

trigone The triangular area at the base of the bladder.

triiodothyronine (T3) A hormone produced by the thyroid gland that helps regulate the body's metabolism.

troponin A cardiac enzyme found in the cells of the heart.

tuberculosis (TB) An airborne infection caused by *Mycobacterium tuberculosis,* bacteria that attack the lungs.

tubulointerstitial nephritis An inflammation of the renal tubules and spaces between the tubules.

tumor An abnormal growth of cells or tissues.

two-pillow orthopnea A description of the patient's sleep habits in which the patient requires two pillows to breathe comfortably while sleeping.

tympanoplasty The surgical repair of the eardrum (tympanic membrane) or bones of the middle ear.

Tzanck test A method of testing skin sores for the herpes simplex virus or varicella zoster virus.

U

ulcerative colitis An ulcerated inflammation of the top layer of the large intestine.

ulna One of two forearm bones, located on the little finger side of the arm.

ultrasound A diagnostic technique that uses high frequency sound waves to create an image of the internal organs.

umbilical cord A cord composed of blood vessels and connective tissue that is connected to the fetus from the placenta.

upper gastrointestinal (GI) series, syn. barium swallow An x-ray examination of the esophagus, stomach, and duodenum using contrast material.

upper respiratory tract The part of the respiratory system that includes the nose, nasal cavities, sinuses, mouth, and pharynx.

urea A byproduct of the metabolic process in the liver.

uremia, *syn.* **azotemia** An excess of urea and other nitrogenous waste in the blood.

ureterocele When the portion of the ureter closest to the bladder becomes enlarged because the ureter opening is very tiny and obstructs urine outflow, causing urine to back up in the ureter tube.

ureteroscope An optical device that is inserted into the urethra and passed up through the bladder to the ureter in order to inspect the opening of the ureters.

ureters The two narrow tubes that carry urine from the kidneys to the bladder.

urethra The canal leading from the bladder that discharges the urine externally.

urethritis An infection limited to the urethra.

urge incontinence The inability to hold urine long enough to reach a restroom.

urinalysis The laboratory examination of urine for various cells and chemicals, such as red blood cells, white blood cells, infection, or excessive protein.

urinary incontinence The loss of bladder control.

urinary tract infection (UTI) An infection that occurs in the urinary tract often caused by bacteria such as *Escherichia coli.*

uroflowmetry, *syn.* **urine flow study** A urodynamic study in which the patient urinates into a device that measures urine speed and volume.

Urogenital A term referring to the urinary and reproductive systems.

Urolithiasis Another name for *nephrolithiasis.*

Urologist A medical doctor who specializes in treating conditions related to the kidneys and urinary tract, and the genital tract or reproductive system in males.

Urology The branch of medicine concerned with the urinary tract in both genders, and with the genital tract or reproductive system in the male.

urostomy, *syn.* **urinary diversion** A surgical procedure to divert urine flow from its normal pathway out of the body.

urticaria, *syn.* **hives** A rash of round, red, itchy welts on the skin.

uterine artery embolization A procedure that blocks the blood vessels that supply a uterine fibroid by injecting small particles of polyvinyl alcohol (PVA) into the arteries that supply it.

uterine cancer Cancer that originates in the body and muscle layers of the uterus.

uterine fibroids, *syn.* **myomas or leiomyomas** Noncancerous growths composed of muscle and fibrous tissue located in or on the uterus.

uterine sarcoma A cancer that originates in the myometrium of the uterus.

uterus, *syn.* **Womb** A pear-shaped organ located in the middle of the pelvis that holds and nourishes a growing fetus.

Uveitis An inflammation of any portion of the uveal tract, which is the middle layer of the eye between the retina and sclera.

Uvula A small piece of soft tissue hanging down from the soft palate over the back of the tongue, which is used primarily in speech production.

V

vacuum extractor A suction device used to assist with delivery of an infant.

vagina, *syn.* **birth canal** A muscular tube projecting inside a female that connects the uterus to the outside of the body.

vaginal atrophy The drying and thinning of the tissues of the vagina and urethra typically seen in menopause which can lead to dyspareunia (pain during sexual intercourse) as well as vaginitis, cystitis, and urinary tract infections.

vaginal hysterectomy A hysterectomy performed by means of access through the vagina.

vaginal wet mount, *syn.* **vaginal smear** A test performed on a sample of vaginal discharge to check for micro-organisms which may have caused an infection.

vagotomy The surgical cutting of the vagus nerve adjacent to the esophagus in order to reduce acid secretions in the stomach.

vagus nerve The cranial nerve that helps control function of the esophagus, larynx, stomach, intestines, lungs, and heart.

Valsalva maneuver A maneuver that increases pressure in the nasopharynx, forcing air into the eustachian tube as all other outlets are blocked.

valve In the heart, the structures that open and close with each heartbeat to ensure the proper sequence of blood flow through the heart.

vasculature The network of blood vessels associated with a particular organ.

vasculitis An inflammation of the blood vessels and the different disorders that can result therefrom.

vasoconstriction The constriction of the smooth muscle in an artery wall that causes the artery to become smaller in diameter.

vasodilation The relaxation of the smooth muscle in an artery wall that causes the artery to become larger in diameter.

vasodilators Drugs that improve blood flow to vessels by dilating them.

vegetation An abnormal growth named for its similarity to natural growth of organic vegetation. In cardiology, this term relates to irregular growths of platelets, fibrin and bacteria on the valves of the heart, causing scarring and narrowing.

vein A vessel that carries oxygen-depleted blood back to the heart.

vena cava filter A device inserted inside the inferior vena cava to catch clots as they try to move through the body to the lungs.

venereal diseases An outdated term for *sexually transmitted diseases*.

ventilation The exchange of air between the lungs and the atmosphere so that oxygen can be exchanged for carbon dioxide at the alveoli.

ventilator A machine that mechanically assists the patient in the exchange of oxygen and carbon dioxide.

ventricles of the brain A network of four chambers in the brain that produce cerebrospinal fluid (CSF).

ventricles of the heart The lower chambers of the heart that collect blood from the right and left atria and pump it out of the heart to the rest of the body.

ventricular fibrillation An abnormal irregular heart rhythm whereby there are very rapid uncoordinated fluttering contractions of the ventricles of the heart, resulting in the disruption between the synchrony of the heartbeat and the pulse.

ventricular septal defect (VSD) A hole in the wall that separates the ventricles of the heart.

ventricular tachycardia A fast heart rhythm that originates in one of the ventricles of the heart.

ventriculoperitoneal (VP) shunt A shunt placed inside one of the ventricles of the brain; its other end is placed into the abdominal cavity.

ventriculostomy A surgical opening made between two ventricles to allow flow of CSF to be unobstructed.

venules Small vessels that gather blood from the capillaries; these venules, in turn, drain into the larger veins that carry deoxygenated blood back to the heart.

Veress needle A special needle used to pump carbon dioxide (CO2) into the abdomen to separate the organs inside the abdominal cavity during surgery.

vermiform appendix A narrow, finger-like tube attached to the cecum that has no real function.

Verrucae Also called *warts*, small, noncancerous skin growths caused by the papillomavirus.

vertebrae (singular *vertebra*) The bones of the spine.

vertebral column The stack of small bones (vertebrae) that make up the spine.

Vertigo A sensation of dizziness as a result of a disorder or blockage in the structures of the inner ear.

vesicoureteral reflux (VUR) The abnormal flow of urine from the bladder back into the ureters; often as a result of a urinary tract infection or birth defect.

vesicular A term that describes breath sounds that are normal.

vestibular organs The utricle, saccule, and semicircular canals located in the inner ear, which help maintain the body's sense of balance.

vestibular system The sensory system involved in maintaining the body's equilibrium.

video EEG An EEG test used to record seizures as they occur.

viral hepatitis An invasion of the liver by one of several hepatitis viruses that infect the liver and begin replicating, delineated by types (A, B, C, D, and E).

viral load The level of HIV in the circulating blood.

viral meningitis A virus infection that causes inflammation of the meninges.

visceral layer Inner layer of the pleura.

viscus (plural **viscera**) The internal organs in the main cavities of the body, especially those in the abdomen, such as the intestines.

visual acuity The ability to perceive detail (acuity), color and contrast, and to distinguish objects.

visual field The total area in which objects can be seen, without moving the head or eye.

visual field testing Diagnostic tests that are used to determine areas of impaired or absent vision due to an ocular or neurologic abnormality.

vitrectomy A procedure performed to remove the vitreous and replace it with a salt solution.

vitreous humor A jelly-like, colorless, transparent substance occupying the greater part of the cavity of the eye, and all the space between the crystalline lens and the retina.

vocal cord paralysis The inability of one or both vocal folds (vocal cords) to move because of damage to the brain or nerves.

vocal cords, *syn.* **vocal folds** Muscular folds of mucous membrane that extend from the laryngeal wall, enclosed in elastic ligament and muscles that control the tension and rate of vibration of the cords as air passes through them to create sounds.

voluntary muscle A muscle whose movement is controlled by the cerebral motor cortex and the cerebellum of the brain.

V/Q scan, *syn.* **ventilation-perfusion scan** A scan used to assess distribution of blood flow and ventilation throughout both lungs.

Vulva The area in which the female external genitalia organs are found.

W

walking pneumonia A type of pneumonia caused by the bacterium *Mycoplasma pneumoniae*, which is a pneumonia that is not severe enough for an infected person to become bedridden or hospitalized.

waveform The visual representation of each electrical impulse detected by leads during an EKG/ECG.

wean (from ventilator) To withdraw or remove the breathing machine so that the patient can breathe independently.

wedge resection Removal of part of a lobe of the lung.

wet mount A test in which a sample of body fluid is examined under the microscope for the presence of microorganisms.

Wheezes Airy, whistling-type sounds made on exhalation.

Y

yellow marrow Bone marrow that does not have any blood-producing function but serves as a storage site for fat cells.

INDEX

Page numbers in bold type refer to illustrations.